AF848793

DENTISTRY AND ORAL SCIENCES

SORT PROGRAMME

A STRUCTURED ORTHODONTIC RESIDENT'S TRAINING PROGRAMME

DENTISTRY AND ORAL SCIENCES

Additional books and e-books in this series can be found on Nova's website under the Series tab.

DENTISTRY AND ORAL SCIENCES

SORT PROGRAMME

A STRUCTURED ORTHODONTIC RESIDENT'S TRAINING PROGRAMME

AMJAD MAHMOOD, BDS, FDS RCSEd (UK)

PROFESSOR OF ORTHODONTICS
PRINCIPAL AND DEAN, MARGALLA COLLEGE OF DENTISTRY
CHIEF ADMINISTRATOR,
MARGALLA INSTITUTE OF HEALTH SCIENCES
RAWALPINDI, PAKISTAN

ROZINA NAZIR, BDS, FCPS, MHPE

ASSOCIATE DEAN CLINICAL SCIENCES
PROFESSOR AND HEAD, DEPARTMENT OF ORTHODONTICS
FOUNDATION UNIVERSITY COLLEGE OF DENTISTRY AND HOSPITAL
ISLAMABAD, PAKISTAN

nova
Medicine & Health
New York

Copyright © 2020 by Nova Science Publishers, Inc.

All rights reserved. No part of this book may be reproduced, stored in a retrieval system or transmitted in any form or by any means: electronic, electrostatic, magnetic, tape, mechanical photocopying, recording or otherwise without the written permission of the Publisher.

We have partnered with Copyright Clearance Center to make it easy for you to obtain permissions to reuse content from this publication. Simply navigate to this publication's page on Nova's website and locate the "Get Permission" button below the title description. This button is linked directly to the title's permission page on copyright.com. Alternatively, you can visit copyright.com and search by title, ISBN, or ISSN.

For further questions about using the service on copyright.com, please contact:
Copyright Clearance Center
Phone: +1-(978) 750-8400 Fax: +1-(978) 750-4470 E-mail: info@copyright.com.

NOTICE TO THE READER

The Publisher has taken reasonable care in the preparation of this book, but makes no expressed or implied warranty of any kind and assumes no responsibility for any errors or omissions. No liability is assumed for incidental or consequential damages in connection with or arising out of information contained in this book. The Publisher shall not be liable for any special, consequential, or exemplary damages resulting, in whole or in part, from the readers' use of, or reliance upon, this material. Any parts of this book based on government reports are so indicated and copyright is claimed for those parts to the extent applicable to compilations of such works.

Independent verification should be sought for any data, advice or recommendations contained in this book. In addition, no responsibility is assumed by the publisher for any injury and/or damage to persons or property arising from any methods, products, instructions, ideas or otherwise contained in this publication.

This publication is designed to provide accurate and authoritative information with regard to the subject matter covered herein. It is sold with the clear understanding that the Publisher is not engaged in rendering legal or any other professional services. If legal or any other expert assistance is required, the services of a competent person should be sought. FROM A DECLARATION OF PARTICIPANTS JOINTLY ADOPTED BY A COMMITTEE OF THE AMERICAN BAR ASSOCIATION AND A COMMITTEE OF PUBLISHERS.

Additional color graphics may be available in the e-book version of this book.

Library of Congress Cataloging-in-Publication Data

ISBN: 978-1-53617-007-8

Published by Nova Science Publishers, Inc. † New York

Dedication

To My parents, who struggled for whatever I am,
My wife & children, who suffered for whatever I am
and
Myself, who had to struggle and suffer

Amjad Mahmood

This Book is dedicated, with all my love and thanks,
to My Parents, My Husband and My Son
who have been a source of strong support, encouragement
and appreciation in my life and career

Rozina Nazir

CONTENTS

Foreword		**ix**
	Derek Mahony	
Preface		**xiii**
Acknowledgments		**xv**
Abbreviations		**xvii**
Chapter 1	Introduction	**1**
Chapter 2	General Instructions	**3**
Chapter 3	Knowledge	**7**
Chapter 4	Skills	**11**
Chapter 5	Attitudes	**13**
Chapter 6	Some Important Points	**15**
Chapter 7	Criteria For Fitness to Appear in Exit Examination	**17**
Chapter 8	Module-I	**19**
Chapter 9	Module-II	**27**
Chapter 10	Module III	**35**
Chapter 11	Module-IV	**45**

Chapter 12	Intermediate Exam (At the Completion of Modules I-IV)	**53**
Chapter 13	Module-V	**55**
Chapter 14	Module-VI	**63**
Chapter 15	Module-VII	**71**
Chapter 16	Module-VIII	**77**
Chapter 17	Exit Exam (At the Completion of Modules I-VIII)	**85**
Chapter 18	BI-Annual Review Proforma (B-ARP)	**87**
Chapter 19	Sample of Schedules	**91**
Chapter 20	Sample of Weekly Time Table	**93**
Chapter 21	List of Logistics for Residents	**95**
Chapter 22	Annexures	**97**
Chapter 23	Log Book	**141**
References		**249**
Index		**255**
About This Book		**261**

FOREWORD

It is an honour to pen the foreword of this book "SORT Programme, A Structured Orthodontic Resident Training Programme". This wonderfully coordinated team effort of both the authors, who are academician, as well as clinicians, appropriately brings in a fine curriculum outline for the postgraduate students in orthodontics. This curriculum covers all the aspects of postgraduate training.

The history of establishing a curriculum in orthodontics goes back to 1961, when the minimal educational requirements for the specialty were formulated in the United States. This book will provide the reader with all aspects of graduate training, within orthodontics, including guidelines for continuing further education. Even though the first schools in orthodontics opened in St. Louis Missouri, more than a hundred years ago, a formulised curriculum was not laid down until 1961, on the understanding that the basic dental degree did not prepare a general dentist sufficiently to practice in the field of orthodontics, and dentofacial orthopedics.

In Europe, the Erasmus project guidelines were first publicised in 1992, and then updated in 2014. I am pleased to say that this book has reviewed both the Erasmus guidelines, as well as those of the American

Orthodontic Association, before formulating its own individualised curriculum.

In Pakistan, the orthodontic specialisation, despite a rigorous four year training for degree requirement, has been successful in attracting the largest groups in residency. This SORT programme is designed in such a way that it will help these residents to be trained to the required standards, in a methodical way.

Curriculum in the past, had classified an Orthodontist, based on the technique they were exposed to. We must all realise that for treatment to be successful, it should be goal orientated, and patient focused, rather than being bound by a specific technique. The graduate training programme, outlined in this book, covers several treatment approaches, and the formulation of a treatment plan based on a solid knowledge of both biology and biomechanics.

As an Orthodontist, with 30 years' experience, I note that year by year, there is a growing population of adult patients, who require orthodontics as part of an overall rehabilitation, which may include periodontal treatment, as well as prosthodontics. This is why an orthodontic graduate need to possess knowledge of the aging process, and the influence of general diseases on the periodontium and the bone. These new orthodontic graduates will have a much greater interaction with other specialties, and other disciplines, as the older the patient, the more interdisciplinary treatment may be required.

This book has four sections. The first section consists of basic information like how to use this programme. The second section has details of all the eight modules, which an orthodontic resident has to undertake in four years of training. Every Module has five important segments: Learning Objectives, Areas to be covered in the module, Reading list, Table Of Specifications, Assessment method and Checklist. The third section is comprised of annexures which contain specific evaluation proformas for Mini-CEX, CbD, OOT, PPP and DOPS. The last part of the textbook consists of logbook to be covered in Module I and II.

We should also emphasise that our profession must remain as one of the leaders in scientific research. It is important to understand that a good solid orthodontic education is only one component. After graduation, we encourage an orthodontic resident to continue to promote at the specialty, and conduct clinical based research. I have found more satisfaction gained by coming up with solutions, to difficult problems, such as Pediatric OSA, rather than just appliance driven orthodontics. I would like to summarise by saying that this book outlines State of the Art education, and future possibilities in training. We should also keep in mind that our profession is there for the benefit of our patients, and anything we can do to contribute to the betterment of our profession via research, and patient focused treatment plans, will also benefit the profession, as a whole.

Dr. Derek Mahony
Registered Specialist in Orthodontics
BDS (Syd), MSc Orth (Lon), D OrthRCS (Edin),
MDOrth RCPS (Glas),
MOrth RCS (Eng), FRCD (Can), MOrth RCS (Edin), FICD, IBO,
FACD, FICCDE, FIADFE, FPFA, Grad Dip Dental Sleep Medicine
(WA), Grad Dip Dent (Ortho)
Diplomate of the International Board of Orthodontics

PREFACE

This curriculum, in its original form, was made for postgraduate training in orthodontics at KRL Hospital, Islamabad by the first author and was in use since 2004. During an MHPE session at the University of Health Sciences, Lahore, the authors were tasked to make an assessment plan for a study module/training programme and it was thought pertinent to use the orthodontic postgraduate training programme as a model. The authors later took the task further and changed the entire programme. Currently, the programme is in use for FCPS/MCPS courses (of the College of Physicians & Surgeons of Pakistan) at the Margalla Institute of Health Sciences, Rawalpindi and is equally useful for other programmes spanning the same duration.

This programme, in its current shape, was prepared in 2014 and published in Pakistan Orthodontic Journal. Since its full implementation in January 2015, many changes have been incorporated in the programme. A dedicated reading list has been added to each module. Specified proformas for each assessment tool were constructed and are attached here as annexures. Certain segments have been redistributed among the modules. Moreover, all the contents of the checklist have been distributed month-wise in each module. To assess the trainees' performance of patients' treatment progress, the Patient Progress

Proforma (PPP) has also been devised. In addition to these, the entire programme has been refined and fine-tuned after multiple feedbacks from assessors and assesses. This book is a result of extensive team work over the past six years. Mere compilation of the data in the form of a book took around one complete year. It is published here for two purposes: for benefit and use of institutions running programmes of matching durations and for continuous improvement and evaluation of the programme by inviting input from every corner.

The programme has been devised in a structured format, whereby, the whole training is patient-centered and follows the actual treatment sequence. Module-I is about activation of prior knowledge of basic medical and dental sciences and attainment of basic clinical knowledge and skills to prepare the residents for an empathetic patient care. Real patient encounter starts in Module-II and from here onwards, all areas of respective modules are according to treatment requirements at different stages.

Each module has six distinct areas, i.e., Learning Objectives, Topics Covered, Reading List, Table of Specifications, Assessment Methods and Check List.

Successful adoption of this modular form of teaching should result in residents attaining the appropriate knowledge, proper attitudes and basic skills required in orthodontics. It additionally enables residents to gain knowledge about medical ethics and develop a sense of professionalism, a scientific attitude and an inquisitive mind, and instill in them, a quest for research and continuing professional development. A modular form of postgraduate training in orthodontics is proposed with an intention to standardize orthodontic training across the country.

Amjad Mahmood
Rozina Nazir

ACKNOWLEDGMENTS

We would like to express our appreciation to Dr. Sirajul Haque Shaikh Director DME, College of Physicians & Surgeons Pakistan for his valuable feedback on this programme. We are grateful to Dr. Kausar Ilyas and Dr. Mehwish Shaheed of Orthodontic department of Margalla College for helping us in making and running of weekly schedule, for their role as co-assessors, in compiling of modular results and their constant feedback. Our special thanks to Dr. Kanwal Zulfiqar of Islamic International Medical & Dental College, Islamabad for her major contribution in writing of reading list of each module.

We also owe many thanks to our residents for their input about the programme since its piloting in 2014, especially Dr. Zainab Hayat, Dr. Hadia Arshad and Dr. Maleeha Mumtaz. Finally, we would like to thank Dr. Tania Arshad for her help in fine tuning of the book.

ABBREVIATIONS

AM	Assessment Method
A	Attitudes
B-ARP	Bi-Annual Review Proforma
CbD	Case based Discussion
CL	Checklist
CIT	Critical Incident Technique
DOPS	Direct Observation of Procedural Skills
EOM	End Of Module
IS	Instructional Strategies
JCM	Journal Club Meeting
K	Knowledge
LOs	Learning Objectives
LCC	Long Clinical Case
Mini-CEX	Mini-Clinical Evaluation Exercise
MCQ	Multiple Choice Question
OOT	Observation Of Teaching
PPP	Patient Progress Proforma
PAL	Peer Assisted Learning
S	Skills
SAQ	Short Answer Question

SCC	Short Clinical Case
TOS	Table of Specifications
TOACS	Task Oriented Assessment of Clinical Skills
WPBA	Workplace-Based Assessment

Chapter 1

INTRODUCTION

The whole programme is divided into VIII modules of six months each and the syllabus for postgraduate orthodontics is distributed in these [1]. The modules are structured in line with the basic learning theories that encompass knowledge, skills and attitudes to be integral to learning of any individual. Keeping in view the Bloom's taxonomy, the learning areas are divided in three domains of Knowledge (K), Skills (S) and Attitudes (A) [2]. The Learning Objectives (LOs) and Instructional Strategies are according to the individual needs of each area and specific tools of assessment are used for every segment of learning (shown in the Table of Specifications, TOS). It is mandatory for the trainees to pass each segment (K, S & A) individually. This separation ensures coverage of all areas especially the affective domain, which otherwise gets neglected. The study topics (Knowledge i.e., cognitive domain) for each module cover a certain area of the curriculum and the trainees have to study these through weekly Peer Assisted Learning (PAL) [3], Presentations, Journal Club Meetings (JCM) and self-study. Using the PAL technique, the senior residents teach the immediate junior batch. In the JCM, the relevant articles from the past and present journals, related to the study topics, are discussed. The Skills (psychomotor skills) and Attitudes (affective domain) are synchronous with the study topics and distributed in each module.

The scoring of each division (K, S & A) is done separately. The knowledge is assessed by scoring of weekly PAL, JCM and Presentation sessions. These scorings are done by the Observation Of Teaching (OOT) proforma. The scores of all these sessions are added. The End Of Module (EOM) exam for Knowledge, comprises of Multiple Choice Questions (MCQs) and Short Answer Questions (SAQs) while Viva questions are incorporated in Task Oriented Assessment of Clinical Skills (TOACS). The assessment tools of Workplace-Based Assessment (WPBA) [4], along with the Checklist (CL) are used for the assessment of Skills and Attitudes. These include Mini-Clinical Evaluation Exercise (Mini-CEX), Direct Observation of Procedural Skills (DOPS), Case based Discussion (CbD) [5], Patient Progress Proforma (PPP) and OOT. The Critical Incident Technique (CIT) [6] is used for scoring of individuals happening of one of its kind. The scores of all these assessment tools are added. The EOM exam for Skills and Attitudes include TOACS, MCQ, SAQ, Short Clinical Case (SCC), and Long Clinical Case (LCC).

As per Wilkinson "WPBA may be part of formative or summative assessment; the former checks progress and informs the educational process, whereas the latter checks what the student has achieved and 'knows how/can do' what the course learning outcomes entailed [7]." The assessment tools are constructed in such a manner that they can be used for formative, summative or a combination of both assessments. The authors prefer a combination of formative and summative assessments. Verbal Feedback is mandatory at the end of each session which substantially aids in the learning process. The cumulative score of the six-monthly module is used for promotion to the next module and 60% score is the bare minimum requirement for that. The entire collection of WPBA of each module forms the Bi-Annual Review Proforma (B-ARP) [8]. The assessment Proforma's for OOT, DOPS, Mini-CEX, CbD, PPP and CL, etc. are attached at the end in Annexures.

Chapter 2

GENERAL INSTRUCTIONS

2.1. This Structured training program is meant for postgraduate training in orthodontics. All the content is covered in 4 years, which is divided into VIII modules. Each module lasts for 6 months. First IV modules are structured in a way that they can be used for any 2 years training programme. Evaluation of trainees is based on WPBA, carried out during the module and an EOM Exam.

2.2. Each module consists of 3 components; K, S & A. The LOs and instructional strategies for K, S & A are mentioned in each module. The assessment of each component is done separately. Assessor can be a Supervisor, Co- Supervisor, Potential Supervisor or a Senior Registrar. The knowledge is assessed by OOT Proforma for presentation, JCM, PAL during the module and by MCQs, SAQs and Viva questions (incorporated in TOACS) taken during EOM examination. Skills and Attitudes are assessed by CbD, CL, PAL and PPP, each done on monthly basis. Skills and Attitudes are also assessed on bimonthly basis by DOPS, Mini-CEX, Presentation and JCM. They are further assessed, once in each module, by OOT for Lecture/ Demonstration during the module and by TOACS, LCC and SCCs during EOM examination.

2.3. The specimen Proforma for OOT, PPP, Mini-CEX, DOPS, etc. are given at the end in annexures. PAL, Presentation, Lecture/ Demonstrations and JCM are marked on OOT. They are constructed in such a manner that they can be used for formative as well as summative assessment. For formative assessment, they can be used on the given scale which has five levels, i.e., 1-Below Expectation, 2-Border line, 3-Meets expectations, 4-Good and 5–Excellent. For summative assessment marks can be allocated (as preferred by the authors) for each level as 2, 4 6, 8 and 10 respectively.

2.4. It is mandatory to cover all the content of a module and get a cumulative score of 60% in each component (K, S & A) separately. The trainee can reappear in failed/weak segment during the same module with the consent of his/her assessor and achieve the required standard. After the compilation of B-ARP, the failed component (K, S, A) is reassessed as follows;

   2.4.1. The Knowledge is reassessed by taking a supplementary exam.

   2.4.2. The Trainee needs to reappear only in the failed component of Skills and Attitudes (CbD, DOPS, Mini-CEX, OOT, PPP, etc.) during the next module and they are reassessed preferably by the same assessor.

2.5. The trainees have to attend four mandatory workshops during Module II. These are Research Methodology, Biostatistics and Dissertation Writing, Communication skills, Introduction to computer and internet and Basic Life Support.

2.6. In order to get promoted to next module the trainee has to complete all the CL during the same module.

2.7. It is mandatory for the trainee to pass the failed component of Modules I, II, III, V, VI & VII in the succeeding module, otherwise the trainee stays in the succeeding module for at least six months and completes the deficiencies. In case of deficient CL and incomplete Synopsis/Dissertation/Research paper 1/Research paper 2 found at the compilation of B-ARP, the remedial action is possible till the end of next module only.

2.8. However, in case of failure in Module IV & VIII, the trainee stays in the same module for another six months till he or she passes each component (K, S & A) plus fulfils all the requirements of “Fitness to appear in Exit Examination” described at the end of the sections.

Chapter 3

KNOWLEDGE

The study topics for each module cover a certain area of the curriculum and the trainees have to study these through PAL and self-study. The other instructional strategies used are weekly Presentations and JCM. Using weekly PAL session, the senior residents teach the immediate junior batch. In the JCM, the articles from the latest journals, related to the study topics, are discussed.

3.1. PAL:

3.1.1. Each month one PAL session is scored, according to an OOT Proforma, by the assessor who observes the whole activity. The presenters are assessed on the basis of their presentation and the attendees are assessed on the basis of their active participation and receptiveness.

3.1.2. Immediate feedback is given by the supervisor and the trainees are informed about their scoring at the end of the session.

3.1.3. Attendance in the PAL is mandatory. Any absentee is marked zero for that session.

3.1.4. Scores for the entire PAL sessions assessed are added for the whole module.

3.2. Presentation:

3.2.1. Topics of presentations are divided among the trainees at the commencement of the module.

3.2.2. One presentation is scored after every two months, according to an OOT Proforma, on the basis of content and delivery of presentation by the presenter. The participants are assessed on the basis of their participation.

3.2.3. Immediate feedback is given by the supervisor and the participants are informed about their scoring at the end of session.

3.2.4. Attendance in the Presentation is mandatory. Any absentee is marked zero for that session.

3.2.5. Scores for all the presentations assessed are added for the whole module.

3.3. JCM:

3.3.1. All trainees are required to prepare the assigned article. Any trainee is chosen randomly, on the day of JCM, to present the article.

3.3.2. After every two months, one JCM is scored, according to an OOT Proforma, on the basis of content and delivery of presentation by the presenter. The participants are assessed on the basis of their active participation.

3.3.3. Immediate feedback is given by the supervisor and the participants are informed about their scoring at the end of session.

3.3.4. Attendance in the JCM is mandatory. Any absentee is marked zero for that session.

3.3.5. Scores for all the JCMs assessed are added for the whole module.

Chapter 4

SKILLS

4.1. The trainees are required to complete the required number of skill tasks in every module (as mentioned in the TOS and CL). The skills are assessed by CbD, Mini-CEX, DOPS, CL, OOT, PPP, TOACS, LCC and SCCs.

4.2. The presenter and attendees are scored during the diagnosis and treatment planning session according to CbD Proforma. Residents in module I will be marked for their diagnostic skills, while from module II and onwards they will be assessed for their treatment planning abilities also. History taking skills are assessed by Mini-CEX. DOPS are used for assessment of clinical procedural skills while CL is used for assessment of non-clinical skills. OOT Proforma is used for assessment of teaching skills during PAL, Presentation, JCM and Lecture/Demo. Patients' progress is assessed by PPP.

4.3. Immediate feedback is given by the assessor and the participants are informed about their scoring at the end of the session. Scores for all the sessions assessed are added for the whole module.

4.4. The skills are assessed during and at the end of the module and a cumulative score of 60% is mandatory to get promoted to the next module.

4.5. To inculcate research skills, 2 publications in indexed journals are made mandatory for every trainee of modules IV and VIII. This is apart from mandatory Dissertation/Thesis.

Chapter 5

ATTITUDES

5.1. The attitudes are assessed by Mini-CEX, DOPS, PPP, OOT, TOACS and LCC.

5.2. Duties of academic & administrative nature can be assigned to any trainee at any time.

5.3. Trainees are assessed for patient follow-up appointments and timely completion of cases by monthly PPP.

5.4. The CIT is used for scoring of individuals happening of one of its kind.

Chapter 6

Some Important Points

6.1. Patients are allotted at the start of Module II, therefore the "comprehensive case records" is not mentioned in the Skills section of Module I. It is included in Module II through Module IV. At the end of Module IV, residents are not allotted new patients so in Module V again, the "Comprehensive case records" is not mentioned. During Module VI, early started cases are in debonding stage, so from Module VI onward "comprehensive case records" of debonded cases is mentioned. Comprehensive case record assessment duration is from Module II to IV during which new patients/cases are allotted and from Module VI onwards with debonding of early cases.

6.2. After the residents are allotted cases, they start initial orthodontics including bonding and banding in the Module II. From Module III onward they are doing full-fledged orthodontics hence the "comprehensive orthodontics" is mentioned first time in the Module III in Skills section and it appears till the module VIII.

6.3. The number of items to be assessed is flexible. The cumulative score of 60% is kept as a bare minimum to pass a module and is calculated according to the number of items assessed that can vary depending on the number of supervisors, number of residents and work load.

6.4. As an example, a schedule of Module I is given as Annexure at the end of program. It has been designed as per requirements of the current center, however the number of items, assessor and assessees can be modified according to the individual needs and requirements of each centre.

6.5. The LOs, Content to be covered, Instructional Strategies (IS), Assessment Method (AM), Reading list, CL and TOS are mentioned in each module

Chapter 7

CRITERIA FOR FITNESS TO APPEAR IN EXIT EXAMINATION

7.1. After Two Years (Module IV)

7.1.1. Completed two years of training

7.1.2. Completion of Checklist

7.1.3. End of Module IV examination passed

7.1.4. Mandatory Workshops attended

7.1.5. Two Comprehensive Orthodontic cases completed

7.1.6. Research Paper 1 accepted for publication

7.1.7. Synopsis for dissertation/thesis approved by examining body

7.2. After Four Years (Module VIII)

7.2.1. Completed four years of training

7.2.2. Completion of Checklist

7.2.3. Certificate of attendance of mandatory workshops

7.2.4. End of Module VIII examination passed

7.2.5. Completed five cases of different variety

7.2.6. Research Paper 2 accepted for publication

7.2.7. Dissertation/Thesis approved by examining body.

Chapter 8

MODULE-I

LEARNING OBJECTIVES

By the end of the module, the trainee should be able to;

- Explain cell, molecular biology, genetics and normal & abnormal growth of craniofacial region.
- Identify significance of medical and oral pathological conditions in orthodontic diagnosis and incorporate it appropriately
- Perform and interpret basic diagnostic record.
- Perform the basic wire work.
- Demonstrate ability to counsel patient, obtain consent and preserve patient privacy and confidentiality.

Module-I: Topics to be Covered

Knowledge			Skills and Attitudes			
Knowledge (K)	**Instructional Strategies (K)**	**Assessment Items (K)**	**Skills (S)**	**Attitudes (A)**	**Instructional Strategies (S &A)**	**Assessment Items (S &A)**

• Cell, molecular biology, genetics, embryology, growth and development
• Patient behaviour, psychology & motivation
• Craniofacial anomalies/ syndromes, cleft lip and palate (basic knowledge)
• Orthodontic diagnosis: (development of problem list)
• Medical conditions related to dentistry
• Oral pathology
	• Self-study
	• Peer Assisted Learning (PAL) {lectures by second year residents}
	• Weekly presentation
	• Weekly journal club meeting (JCM)
		• End of module exam comprising of MCQs, SAQs, Viva
		• OOT (PAL)
		• OOT (Presentation)
		• OOT (JCM)
			• Ceph tracing & Analysis (log book)
			• Impression taking, wax bite and model trimming
			• Photography
			• History taking
			• Cast analysis including mixed dentition & Bolton analysis
			• Orthodontic Diagnostic skills
			• Wire work (5 Each)
			  • Finger spring
			  • Z-spring
			  • T-spring
			  • Canine retractor
			  • Adams clasp
			  • Ball ended clasp
			  • C clasp
			  • Labial bow
			• Feeding Plate (1 each)
			  • For Unilateral cleft
			  • For Bilateral cleft
				• Explaining the procedure before hand
				• Obtain patient's consent
				• Ensure Patient's comfort
				• Maintain privacy of the patient
				• Preserve Confidentiality of the patient
					• Peer Assisted Learning (PAL) (demonstrations by senior residents)
					• Self-practice
						• CbD
						• CL
						• DOPS
						• Mini-CEX
						• TOACS
						• CIT

Module-I: Reading List

	Topic	References
1	**Cell, Molecular Biology, Genetics**	• Textbook of Medical Physiology, Guyton and Hall, 12th Edition- Chapter 2, The cell and its functions • Lippincott's Illustrated Reviews- Biochemistry, 6th Edition- Denise R Ferrier, Unit IV, Chapter 29-33 • Orthodontics Current Principles and Techniques, 6th Edition- Lee W Grabber, Robert L. Vanarsdall Jr, Chapter 2 • Craniofacial Sutures- Development, disease and Treatment- D.P RICE, Genetics of Craniosynostosis: Genes, Syndromes, Mutations and Genotype-Phenotype Correlations • Seminars in Orthodontics, June 2008, Volume 14, Issue 2, Genetics and Orthodontics
2	**Embryology, Growth and Development**	• Essentials of Facial Growth – Donald H. Enlow • Contemporary Orthodontics. 5th edition. William R Proffit, Henry W Fields, David M Sarver, Chapter 2, 3, 4, 5 • Textbook of Orthodontics- Bishara, chapter 1-8 • An Introduction to Orthodontics, 3rd Edition - Laura Mitchel, Chapter 4 • Handbook of Orthodontics-Moyer's, Chapter 2, 3, 4, 5, 6, 7 • Orthodontics Current Principles and Techniques, 6th Edition- Lee W Grabber, Robert L. Vanarsdall Jr, Chapter 1 • Postgraduate Notes in Orthodontics, 5th Edition-Bristol, Growth, Chapter21 • Mosby's Orthodontic review, Chapter 1, 2 • Orthodontic diagnosis- Thomas Rakosi, Thomas M Grabber, Growth of Craniofacial structures 8-33 • Craniofacial Sutures- Development, disease and Treatment- D.P RICE, 1 Developmental Anatomy of Craniofacial Sutures • Seminars in Orthodontics, December 2005, Volume 11, Issue 4, Control Mechanisms of Craniofacial Development and Growth
3	**Patient behaviour, psychology and motivation**	• Contemporary Treatment of Dentofacial Deformity. William R Proffit, Raymond P White, David M Sarver, Chapter 3 • Textbook of Orthodontics- Bishara, 25 • Biomechanics and Esthetic Strategies in Clinical Orthodontics- Ravindra Nanda Chapter 5 • Contemporary Orthodontics. 5th edition. William R Proffit, Henry W Fields, David M Sarver Chapter 2 page 50- 64 • Orthodontics Current Principles and Techniques, 6th Edition- Lee W Grabber, Robert L. Vanarsdall Jr, Chapter 10 • Clinical Problem Solving in Orthodontic and Paediatric Dentistry, Chapter 20
4	**Craniofacial anomalies/ Syndromes, Cleft Lip and Palate**	• Textbook of Orthodontics- Bishara, Chapter 27 • Cleft lip and palate Diagnosis and Management- Sameul Berkowitz • An Introduction to Orthodontics, 3rd Edition - Laura Mitchel, Chapter 22 • Understanding Craniofacial Anomalies- The Etiopathogenesis of Craniosynostoses and Facial Clefting. Mark P. Mooney, Michael Siegel • Contemporary Orthodontics. 5th edition. William R Proffit, Henry W Fields, David M Sarver, Chapter 5, 7 (page 269- 274))

Module-I: Reading List (Continued)

	Topic	References
4	**Craniofacial anomalies/ Syndromes, Cleft Lip and Palate**	• Orthodontics Current Principles and Techniques, 6th Edition- Lee W Grabber, Robert L. Vanarsdall Jr, Chapter 14 • Postgraduate Notes in Orthodontics, 5th Edition-Bristol, Craniofacial anomalies 33 • Craniofacial Sutures- Development, disease and Treatment- D.P RICE, 91 Clinical Features of Syndromic Craniosynostosis • Seminars in Orthodontics, September 1996, Volume 2, Issue 3, p 161-227, Cleft lip and Palate Seminars in Orthodontics, September 2011, Volume 17, Issue 3, p 181-246, Craniofacial Orthodontics II • Orthodontic treatment of Cleft lip and Palate, Birth to adulthood. J Daniel Subtelny. October 1996. (http://www.angle.org/doi/pdf/10.1043/00033219(1966)036%3C0273:OTOCLA%3E2.0.CO%3B2)
5	**Orthodontic Diagnosis**	• Contemporary Orthodontics. 5th edition. William R Proffit, Henry W Fields, David M Sarver, Chapter 6 • Contemporary Treatment of Dentofacial Deformity. William R Proffit, Raymond P White, David M Sarver, Chapter 4, 5 • Orthodontics Current Principles and Techniques, 6th Edition- Lee W Grabber, Robert L. Vanarsdall Jr, Chapter 8, 9, 11, 34 • Postgraduate Notes in Orthodontics, 5th Edition-Bristol, Diagnosis 93 • Textbook of Orthodontics- Bishara, Chapter 9- 13 • Handbook of Orthodontics-Moyer's, Chapter 8, 9, 10, 11, 12 • An Introduction to Orthodontics, 3rd Edition- Laura Mitchel, Chapter 2, 5 • Biomechanics and Esthetic Strategies in Clinical Orthodontics- Ravindra Nanda, Chapter 3 • Facial and Dental planning for Orthodontists and Oral Surgeons- Arnett, Mc Laughlin, Chapter1, 2, 3, 4, 5 • Orthodontic and Orthopaedic treatment in Mixed dentition- James A McNamara, William L Brudon Orthodontic Diagnosis and treatment Planning • Enhancement Orthodontics, Theory and practice- Mark Benard Ackerman, Chapter 3, 4, 5
6	**Medical conditions related to dentistry**	• Contemporary Orthodontics. 5th edition. William R Proffit, Henry W Fields, David M Sarver Chapter 7 page 266-274 • Textbook of Orthodontics- Bishara, Chapter 28 • Postgraduate Notes in Orthodontics, 5th Edition-Bristol, Relevant Medical Disorders 243 • Seminars in Orthodontics, December 2004, Volume 10, Issue 4
7	**Oral pathology**	• Clinical problem solving in Orthodontics and Paediatric Dentistry, Chapter29- 36 • Postgraduate Notes in Orthodontics, 5th Edition-Bristol, Anomalies 75 • Orthodontic diagnosis- Thomas Rikosi, Thomas M Grabber- Etiology of Malocclusion • Contemporary Oral and Maxillofacial Pathology, 2nd Edition- J Philip Sapp, Lewis R. Eversole Chapter 1, 2, 3, 11

Skills		
8	**Wire Bending Skills**	• Contemporary Orthodontics. 5th edition. William R Proffit, Henry W Fields, David M Sarver: Chapter 6, 7 • An Atlas of Removable Orthodontic appliance- Gordon C. Dickson, Albert E. Wheatly.
9	**Cephalometric Tracing & Analysis**	• Radiographic Cephalometry Alaxander Jacobson • Cephalometric Radiography- Thomas Rakosi • A Guide to Cephalometrics- Malcom E Meisttel, Thomas J Cangialosi • Orthodontic and Orthopaedic treatment in Mixed dentition- James A McNamara, William L Brudon Cephalometric Evaluation of Orthodontic Patient
10	**Impression taking, wax bite and model trimming**	• A Modified Technique of Orthodontic Model Trimming- Pakistan Orthodontic Journal, Vol 1, No 1 (2009)
11	**Photography**	• A Short Guide to Clinical Photography in Orthodontics- ShadiSamawi • Orthodontics Current Principles and Techniques, 6th Edition- Lee W Grabber, Robert L. Vanarsdall Jr, Chapter 34 • Orthodontic diagnosis- Thomas Rakosi, Thomas M Grabber Orthodontic records, Case evaluation, Diagnostic procedures
12	**History taking**	• Contemporary Orthodontics. 5th edition. William R Proffit, Henry W Fields, David M Sarver Chapter 6 • Orthodontic diagnosis- Thomas Rakosi, Thomas M Grabber, Orthodontic records, Case evaluation, Diagnostic procedures • Enhancement Orthodontics, Theory and practice- Mark Benard Ackerman, Chapter 2
13	**Cast analysis including mixed dentition & Bolton analysis**	• Contemporary Orthodontics. 5th edition. William R Proffit, Henry W Fields, David M Sarver Chapter 6 • Orthodontics Current Principles and Techniques, 6th Edition- Lee W Grabber, Robert L. Vanarsdall Jr, Chapter 34 • Orthodontic diagnosis- Thomas Rakosi, Thomas M Grabber, Orthodontic records, Case evaluation, Diagnostic procedures
14	**Feeding Plate**	• Presurgical Nasoalveolar Moulding treatment in cleft lip and palate patients- Barry H. Grayson and Pradip R. Shetye.
15	**Journals**	• AJODO, Seminars in Orthodontics, Angles Orthodontist, European Journal of orthodontics, Cochrane Reviews, Classical Articles

Module-I: Table of Specifications

Areas to be covered in this Module	SAQ	MCQ	TOACS	OOT (PAL)	OOT (Presentation)	OOT (JCM)	CL	CbD	Mini-CEX	DOPS
Knowledge (K)										
• Cell, molecular biology, genetics, embryology, growth and development	1	6	1	1	1					
• Craniofacial anomalies/syndromes, cleft lip and palate (basic knowledge)	1	6		1		3				
• Orthodontic diagnosis: (development of problem list)	1	6		1	1		-	-	-	-
• Medical conditions related to dentistry	1	3		1						
• Oral pathology	1	6	1	1						
• Patient behaviour, psychology and motivation	1	3		1	1					
Skills (S)										
• History taking	-	-	1	-	-	-	-	-	3	-
• Ceph tracing & analysis	-	-	1	-	-	-	2	-	-	-
• Model trimming	-	-	-	-	-	-	1	-	-	-
• Photography	-	-	-	-	-	-		-	-	1
• Cast analysis including mixed dentition & Bolton analysis	-	-	-	-	-	-	1	-	-	-
• Feeding Plate	-	-	-	-	-	-	1	-	-	-
• Wire work	-	-	1	-	-	-	1	-	-	-
• Impression taking and wax bite	-	-	-	-	-	-		-	-	2
• Orthodontic Diagnostic Skills	-	-	1	-	-	-		6	-	-
Attitudes (A)										
• Explaining the procedure before hand • Taking consent from the patient • Privacy of the patient • Comfort of the patient • Confidentiality of the patient	-	-	-	-	-	-	-	-	3	3
Total	6	30	6	6	3	3	6	6	6	6

Module I: Assessment Method

Formative + Summative Assessment

During Module by Work Place Based Assessment (WPBA)

Knowledge

1. OOT (PAL)______________6
2. OOT (Presentation)________3
3. OOT (JCM)______________3

Skills + Attitudes

4. CL____________________6
5. CbD__________________6
6. Mini-CEX______________6
7. DOPS_________________6
8. CIT____________________As & when Required

End of Module Examination

Knowledge

9. SAQs_________________6
10. MCQs________________30

Skills + Attitudes

11. TOACS_______________6

Module-I: Checklist

Name of Resident: ______________________

Months	Practical work	Date	Signature of Supervisor
1st Month	Cephalometric Analysis (Log Book first 30 pages)		
2nd Month	Cephalometric Analysis (Log Book Next 30 pages)		
3rd Month	Growth predication Cast Analysis Mixed Dentition Analysis Space Analysis Royal London space Analysis Bolton Analysis ABO Grading & ABO Discrepancy Index IOTN, ICON, PAR Index (Remaining Log Book Module I)		
4th Month	Adam's clasp (5)		
	Labial bow (5)		
	Finger spring (5)		
	T- spring (5)		
5th Month	Ball ended clasp (5)		
	C-clasp (5)		
	Canine retractor (5)		
	Z- spring (5)		
	Feeding plate (2)		
6th Month	Model trimming (1)		
	Photography (1)		
	Synopsis for Research Article 1 approved by the supervisor		

Chapter 9

MODULE-II

LEARNING OBJECTIVES

By the end of the module, the trainee should be able to;

- Apply the knowledge of removable & fixed appliances, development of occlusion, indices and anchorage, etc. to the orthodontic diagnosis and treatment planning.
- Identify the role of mechanics, biomechanics and orthodontic materials in correction of dentofacial anomalies.
- Utilize the knowledge gained from the CPSP workshops pertaining to communication skills, IT & computer technology, research methodology & biostatistics, primary surgical skills and BLS (Basic Life support), etc. for the benefit of orthodontic patients.
- Fabricate appliances related to preventive and interceptive orthodontics.
- Place bands and bond brackets.
- Demonstrate ability to counsel patient, obtain consent and preserve patient privacy and confidentiality
- Exhibit an awareness of protecting self, patient and staff from radiation.

Module-II: Topics to be Covered

Knowledge			Skills and Attitudes			
Knowledge (K)	**Instructional Strategies (K)**	**Assessment Items (K)**	**Skills (S)**	**Attitudes (A)**	**Instructional Strategies (S &A)**	**Assessment Items (S & A)**

• Fixed & Removable appliances
• Development of dentition & occlusion
• Indices
• Timing of orthodontic treatment
• Anchorage
• Preventive & interceptive orthodontics
• Biomechanics & mechanics
• Orthodontic materials
• Radiology and radiography
• Orthodontic diagnosis & treatment planning
• Mandatory Workshops
• TMJ Examination
• Synopsis Writing
	• Self-study
	• Peer Assisted Learning (PAL) {lectures by second year residents}
	• Weekly presentation
	• Weekly journal club meeting (JCM)
		• End of module exam comprising of MCQs, SAQs & Viva
		• OOT (PAL)
		• OOT (Presentation)
		• OOT (JCM)
			• Band cementation & bracket bonding
			• on typodont
			• on patient
			• TPA/Nance button
			• Soldering/welding
			• Orthodontic Diagnostic & Treatment planning skills
			• Preventive & interceptive orthodontic appliances
			  • Space maintainer
			  • Habit breaking appliance
			  • Whip spring
			  • Lip bumper
			  • Oral screen
			  • Mouth guard
			• Hawley's retainer
			• OPG & periapical (taking & interpretation)
			• CBCT (interpretation)
			• Comprehensive case records
			• TMJ Examination
			• Synopsis for Research paper 1
				• Explaining the procedure before hand
				• Obtain patient's consent
				• Ensure Patient's comfort
				• Maintain privacy of the patient
				• Preserve Confidentiality of the patient
				• Radiation safety
					• Peer Assisted Learning (PAL) (demonstration by senior residents)
					• Self-practice
						• CbD
						• CL
						• DOPS
						• Mini-CEX
						• TOACS
						• CIT
						• Submission of synopsis for Research paper 1

Module-II: Reading List

	Topic	References
1	**Fixed and Removable Appliances**	• Contemporary Orthodontics. 5th edition. William R Proffit, Henry W Fields, David M Sarver: Chapter 10, 11, 12, 13, 17 • Orthodontics Current Principles and Techniques, 6th Edition- Lee W Grabber, Robert L. Vanarsdall Jr: Chapter 16, 24, 25, 26, 18, 33, 35 • Orthodontic & Orthopaedic Treatment in Mixed Dentition James A McNamara, William L Brudon: Chapters 7-16, 19 • Invisible orthodontics current concepts and solutions in lingual orthodontics by Giuseppe Scuzzo • Seminar: Lingual orthodontics: The future (Sept 2006) H. Stuart Mc Crostie • An Introduction to Orthodontics, 3rd Edition - Laura Mitchel: Chapters 16, 17 and 18 • Postgraduate Notes in Orthodontics, 5th Edition-Bristol: page 133, 135, 139, 142, 147, 170 • Handbook of Orthodontics-Moyer's: section 18/c, d, e
2	**Development of dentition and occlusion**	• Contemporary Orthodontics. 5th edition. William R Proffit, Henry W Fields, David M Sarver: Chapter 3 • Orthodontics Current Principles and Techniques, 6th Edition- Lee W Grabber, Robert L. Vanarsdall Jr: Chapter 34 • An Introduction to Orthodontics, 3rd Edition- Laura Mitchel: chapter 3 • Management of temporomandibular disorders and occlusion Jeffery P Okeson: Chapter 3 • Handbook of Orthodontics-Moyer's: Chapter 11, 6 • Postgraduate Notes in Orthodontics, 5th Edition-Bristol: pg 48 • Orthodontic & Orthopedic Treatment in Mixed Dentition James A McNamara, William L Brudon: Chapter 3
3	**Indices**	• Postgraduate Notes in Orthodontics, 5th Edition-Bristol: page 99
4	**Timing of orthodontic treatment**	• Contemporary Orthodontics. 5th edition. William R Proffit, Henry W Fields, David M Sarver: Chapter 11, 12, 13 • Orthodontics Current Principles and Techniques, 6th Edition- Lee W Grabber, Robert L. Vanarsdall Jr: Chapter 15, 16, 34 • Orthodontic & Orthopedic Treatment in Mixed Dentition James A McNamara, William L Brudon: chapter 1 • Postgraduate Notes in Orthodontics, 5th Edition-Bristol: page 107
5	**Anchorage**	• Contemporary Orthodontics. 5th edition. William R Proffit, Henry W Fields, David M Sarver: Chapter 8, 9 • Postgraduate Notes in Orthodontics, 5th Edition-Bristol: Chapter anchorage • An Introduction to Orthodontics, 3rd Edition- Laura Mitchel: chapter 15

Module-II: Reading List (Continued)

	Topic	References
6	**Preventive and interceptive orthodontics**	• Contemporary Orthodontics. 5th edition. William R Proffit, Henry W Fields, David M Sarver: Chapter 11, 12, 13 • Orthodontics Current Principles and Techniques, 6th Edition- Lee W Grabber, Robert L. Vanarsdall Jr: chapter 16, 34 • Orthodontic & Orthopedic Treatment in Mixed Dentition James A McNamara, William L Brudon 4, 5, 6 • Handbook of Orthodontics-Moyer's: chapter 15, 16 • Postgraduate Notes in Orthodontics, 5th Edition-Bristol: pg 105
7	**Biomechanics and mechanics**	• Contemporary Orthodontics. 5th edition. William R Proffit, Henry W Fields, David M Sarver: Chapter 8, 9 • Orthodontics Current Principles and Techniques, 6th Edition- Lee W Grabber, Robert L. Vanarsdall Jr: Chapter 3, 4, 5, 17 • Handbook of Orthodontics-Moyer's: chapter 13 • Postgraduate Notes in Orthodontics, 5th Edition-Bristol: theoretical aspect
8	**Orthodontic materials**	• Contemporary Orthodontics. 5th edition. William R Proffit, Henry W Fields, David M Sarver: Chapter 9 • Orthodontics Current Principles and Techniques, 6th Edition- Lee W Grabber, Robert L. Vanarsdall Jr: Chapter 6 • Postgraduate Notes in Orthodontics, 5th Edition-Bristol: pg 203
9	**Radiology and Radiography**	• Contemporary Orthodontics. 5th edition. William R Proffit, Henry W Fields, David M Sarver: Chapter 6 • Orthodontics Current Principles and Techniques, 6th Edition- Lee W Grabber, Robert L. Vanarsdall Jr: Chapter 11 • Postgraduate Notes in Orthodontics, 5th Edition-Bristol: pg 236, 240 • Essentials of dental radiography and Radiology; Eric Waites, Orthodontic diagnosis; Thomas Rakosi • Orthodontic & Orthopedic Treatment in Mixed Dentition James A McNamara, William L Brudon chapter 2
10	**Orthodontic diagnosis and Treatment Planning**	• Contemporary Orthodontics. 5th edition. William R Proffit, Henry W Fields, David M Sarver: Chapter 6, 7 • Orthodontics Current Principles and Techniques, 6th Edition- Lee W Grabber, Robert L. Vanarsdall Jr: Chapter 8, 9, 10 • Handbook of Orthodontics-Moyer's: chapter 8-12 • Postgraduate Notes in Orthodontics, 5th Edition-Bristol: pg 93
11	**Journals**	• AJODO, Seminars in Orthodontics, Angles Orthodontist, European Journal of orthodontics, Cochrane Reviews, Classical Articles

Module-II: Table of Specifications

Areas to be covered in this Module	SAQ	MCQ	TOACS	OOT (PAL)	OOT (Presentation	OOT (JCM)	CL	CbD	Mini-CEX	DOPS
Knowledge (K)										
• Fixed & Removable appliances	1	3	1	1	1	3				
• Development of dentition & occlusion	1	3		1						
• Indices	1	3		1						
• Timing of orthodontic treatment	1	3								
• Anchorage	1	3		1	1					
• Preventive & interceptive orthodontics	1	3	1				-	-	-	-
• Biomechanics & mechanics	1	3		1	1					
• Orthodontic materials	1	3								
• Radiology and Radiography	1	3		1						
• Orthodontic diagnosis & treatment planning	1	3								
Skills (S)										
• Comprehensive Orthodontics	-	-	-	-	-	-	-	-	-	-
• Banding	-	-	-	-	-	-	-	-	-	1
• TMJ Examination	-	-	1	-	-	-	1	-	-	1
• TPA/Nance button/lingual arch	-	-	1	-	-	-	1	-	-	-
• Preventive & interceptive orthodontic appliances (other than TPA Lingual arch	-	-		-	-	-	1	-	-	-
• Orthodontic Diagnostic & Treatment Planning skills	-	-	1	-	-	-	-	6	-	-
• CPG, Lateral ceph & Periapical (taking & interpretation)	-	-	1	-	-	-	-	-	-	1
• CBCT (interpretation)	-	-	1	-	-	-	1	-	-	-
• Hawley's Retainer	-	-	-	-	-	-	1	-	-	-
• Spot welding, Soldering	-	-	1	-	-	-	2	-	-	-
• Comprehensive case records	-	-	-	-	-	-	2	-	3	-
• Synopsis for Research paper 1	-	-	-	-	-	-	1	-	-	-

Module-II: Table of Specifications (Continued)

Areas to be covered in this Module	SAQ	MCQ	TOACS	OOT (PAL)	OOT (Presentation	OOT (JCM)	CL	CbD	Mini-CEX	DOPS
Attitudes (A)										
• Explaining the procedure before hand • Taking consent from the patient • Privacy of the patient • Comfort of the patient • Confidentiality of the patient • Radiation Safety	-	-		-	-	-	-	-	3	3
Total	10	30	8	6	3	3	10	6	6	6

Module-II: Assessment Method

Formative + Summative Assessment

During Module by Work Place Based Assessment (WPBA)

Knowledge

1. OOT (PAL)______________6
2. OOT (Presentation)_______3
3. OOT (JCM)______________3

Skills + Attitudes

4. CL___________________10
5. CbD__________________6
6. Mini-CEX______________6
7. DOPS_________________6
8. CIT___________________As & when Required

End of Module Examination

Knowledge

9. SAQs_________________10
10. MCQs________________30

Skills + Attitudes

11. TOACS________________8

Module-II: Checklist

Name of Resident: ______________________________

Months	Practical work	Date	Signature of Supervisor
1st Month	3-D Digitized landmarks identification & Cephalometric Analysis e.g., View box (Log Book Module-II part)		
	Band cementation Typodont		
	Bracket bonding Typodont		
2nd Month	Comprehensive Case Record (Two)		
	TPA/Nance button fabrication/Lingual arch		
	Soldering/welding (one Each)		
3rd Month	Space maintainer		
	Habit Breaking Appliance		
4th Month	Whip spring		
	Lip bumper		
	Mouth guard		
5th Month	Oral screen		
	Hawley's retainer		
6th Month	CBCT interpretation		
	Submission of Synopsis for Dissertation/Thesis		

Chapter 10

MODULE-III

LEARNING OBJECTIVES

By the end of the module, the trainee should be able to;

- Classify different malocclusions and plan growth modification for skeletal discrepancies in growing children.
- Identify disturbances in dental development and formulate a solution for that problem.
- Fabricate and insert fixed, orthopaedic & expansion appliances, distalizers, headgear, face mask & chin cup, etc.
- Teach the subject of orthodontics & give demonstrations to final year BDS.
- Write synopsis as a prerequisite for dissertation writing.
- Demonstrate insertion of orthodontic mini implant
- Demonstrate basic history taking, examination and diagnostic skills
- Demonstrate ability to counsel patient, obtain consent and preserve patient privacy and confidentiality

Module-III: Topics to be Covered

<table>
<tr><th colspan="3">Knowledge</th><th colspan="4">Skills and Attitudes</th></tr>
<tr><th>Knowledge (K)</th><th>Instructional Strategies (K)</th><th>Assessment Items (K)</th><th>Skills (S)</th><th>Attitudes (A)</th><th>Instructional Strategies (S & A)</th><th>Assessment Items (S & A)</th></tr>
<tr>
<td>• Orthopaedics
• Extra-oral traction
• Arch lengthening & expansion
• Occlusion, oral physiology, malocclusions
• Orthodontic treatment; Phase I (levelling and alignment)
• Disturbances in dental development including impacted teeth
• Smile aesthetics
• Implants
• Teaching & learning
• Ethics and Professionalism</td>
<td>• Self-study
• Peer Assisted Learning (PAL) {lectures by third year residents}
• Weekly presentation
• Weekly journal club meeting (JCM)</td>
<td>• End of module exam comprising of MCQs, SAQs & Viva
• OOT (PAL)
• OOT (Presentation)
• OOT (JCM)</td>
<td>• Comprehensive orthodontics
• Orthodontic Diagnostic & Treatment planning
• Impression, bite registration of functional appliance
• Articulation & fabrication of functional appliances
• Hyrax
• Quad helix
• W-arch
• Nitinol expander
• Bite plates (ant/post)
• Inclined planes
• Molar uprighting and distalizing appliance
• Forsus appliance
• Head gear
• Face mask
• Chin cup
• Implant placement
• Demonstrations & teaching of final year BDS
• Comprehensive case records</td>
<td>• Explaining the procedure before hand
• Obtain patient's consent
• Ensure Patient's comfort
• Maintain privacy of the patient
• Preserve Confidentiality of the patient
• Radiation safety</td>
<td>• Peer Assisted Learning (PAL) (demonstration by senior residents)
• Self-practice</td>
<td>• CbD
• CL
• DOPS
• Mini-CEX
• OOT (Lec/Demo)
• PPP
• TOACS
• CIT</td>
</tr>
</table>

Module-III: Reading List

	Topic	References
1	**Orthopaedics**	• Contemporary Orthodontics. 5th edition. William R Proffit, Henry W Fields, David M Sarver chapter 13: Treatment of skeletal problems in children • Orthodontics Current Principles and Techniques, 6th Edition- Lee W Grabber, Robert L. Vanarsdall Jr chapter 14: Optimizing orthodontic and dentofacial orthopaedic treatment timing, chapter 22: Non-extraction treatment (Headgear) • Postgraduate Notes in Orthodontics, 5th Edition-Bristol: 139-144
2	**Extraoral traction**	• Contemporary Orthodontics. 5th edition. William R Proffit, Henry W Fields, David M Sarver 13: Treatment of skeletal problems in children • Orthodontics Current Principles and Techniques, 6th Edition- Lee W Grabber, Robert L. Vanarsdall Jr Chapter 14: Optimizing orthodontic and dentofacial orthopaedic treatment timing, chapter 22: Non-extraction treatment (Headgear) • Postgraduate Notes in Orthodontics, 5th Edition-Bristol: 139-144
3	**Arch lengthening and expansion**	• Contemporary Orthodontics. 5th edition. William R Proffit, Henry W Fields, David M Sarver chapter 11: Moderate non-skeletal problems in preadolescent children, chapter 12: Complex non-skeletal problems in preadolescent children • Orthodontics Current Principles and Techniques, 6th Edition- Lee W Grabber, Robert L. Vanarsdall Jr chapter 22: Non-extraction treatment • Postgraduate Notes in Orthodontics, 5th Edition-Bristol: 153-157
4	**Occlusion, Oral Physiology, Malocclusion**	• Postgraduate Notes in Orthodontics, 5th Edition-Bristol: 45-74
5	**Orthodontic Treatment: Phase I**	• Contemporary Orthodontics. 5th edition. William R Proffit, Henry W Fields, David M Sarver chapter 14: Levelling and alignment • Orthodontics Current Principles and Techniques, 6th Edition- Lee W Grabber, Robert L. Vanarsdall Jr chapter 16: Straight wire appliance
6	**Disturbances in dental development, Impacted Teeth**	• Contemporary Orthodontics. 5th edition. William R Proffit, Henry W Fields, David M Sarver chapter 12: Complex non-skeletal problems in preadolescent children • Orthodontics Current Principles and Techniques, 6th Edition- Lee W Grabber, Robert L. Vanarsdall Jr (6th edition) chapter 28: Management of impactions • Postgraduate Notes in Orthodontics, 5th Edition-Bristol: 75-92 • Orthodontic treatment of impacted teeth, Adrian Becker

Module-III: Reading List (Continued)

	Topic	References
7	**Smile Aesthetics**	• Contemporary Treatment of Dentofacial Deformity. William R Proffit, Raymond P White, David M Sarver • Contemporary Orthodontics. 5th edition. William R Proffit, Henry W Fields, David M Sarver chapter: Orthodontic diagnosis • Orthodontics Current Principles and Techniques, 6th Edition- Lee W Grabber, Robert L. Vanarsdall Jr chapter 2: Special consideration in diagnosis and treatment planning
8	**Implants**	• Contemporary Orthodontics. 5th edition. William R Proffit, Henry W Fields, David M Sarver chapter 10: Contemporary orthodontic appliances • Orthodontics Current Principles and Techniques, 6th Edition- Lee W Grabber, Robert L. Vanarsdall Jr chapter 12: Biomechanical considerations with TADs • TADs Nanda
9	**Teaching and learning**	• ABC of teaching and learning in Medicine
10	**Ethical Questions in Dentistry**	• JT Rule, RM Veatch, Quintessence, Second Edition 2004, Chapter 4 and Chapter 8 • Ethics Handbook for Dentists American College of Dentists • https://acd.org/PDF/Ethics_Handbook_for_Dentists_(s).pdf
11	**Professionalism**	• Embedding Professionalism In Medical Education Baltimore Maryland as a Tool for Implementation
		Skills
1	**Orthodontic diagnosis and treatment planning skills**	• Contemporary Orthodontics. 5th edition. William R Proffit, Henry W Fields, David M Sarver chapter 6: Orthodontic diagnosis, chapter 7: Orthodontic treatment planning • Orthodontics Current Principles and Techniques, 6th Edition- Lee W Grabber, Robert L. Vanarsdall Jr chapter 1: The decision-making process in orthodontics, chapter 2: Special consideration in diagnosis and treatment planning
2	**Functional appliance**	• Contemporary Orthodontics. 5th edition. William R Proffit, Henry W Fields, David M Sarver chapter 10: Contemporary orthodontic appliances, chapter 13: Treatment of skeletal problems in children • Postgraduate Notes in Orthodontics, 5th Edition-Bristol: 147-152 • Orthodontics Current Principles and Techniques, 6th Edition- Lee W Grabber, Robert L. Vanarsdall Jr chapter 35: Functional appliances
3	**Forsus Appliance**	• Orthodontics Current Principles and Techniques, 6th Edition- Lee W Grabber, Robert L. Vanarsdall Jr chapter 35: Functional appliances

Skills		
4	**Expansion appliances**	• Contemporary Orthodontics. 5th edition. William R Proffit, Henry W Fields, David M Sarver chapter 11: Moderate non-skeletal problems in preadolescent children, chapter 12: Complex non-skeletal problems in preadolescent children • Orthodontics Current Principles and Techniques, 6th Edition- Lee W Grabber, Robert L. Vanarsdall Jr chapter 22: Non-extraction treatment
5	**Molar uprighting and distalizing appliance**	• Contemporary Orthodontics. 5th edition. William R Proffit, Henry W Fields, David M Sarver chapter 18: Special consideration for treatment in adults
6	**Headgear, facemask, chincup**	• Contemporary Orthodontics. 5th edition. William R Proffit, Henry W Fields, David M Sarver chapter 13: Treatment of skeletal problems in children • Orthodontics Current Principles and Techniques, 6th Edition- Lee W Grabber, Robert L. Vanarsdall Jr chapter 14: Optimizing orthodontic and dentofacial orthopaedic treatment timing, chapter 22: Non-extraction treatment (Headgear)
7	**Implant placement**	• Orthodontics Current Principles and Techniques, 6th Edition- Lee W Grabber, Robert L. Vanarsdall Jr chapter 12: Biomechanical considerations with TADs • Temporary Anchorage Devices in Orthodontics Ravindra Nanda
8	**Journals**	• AJODO, Seminars in Orthodontics, Angles Orthodontist, European Journal of orthodontics, Cochrane Reviews, Classical Articles

Module-III: Table of Specifications

Areas to be covered in this Module	SAQ	MCQ	TOACS	OOT (PAL)	OOT (Presentation)	OOT (JCM)	OOT (Lec/ Demo)	CL	CbD	Mini-CEX	DOPS	PPP
Knowledge (K)												
• **Orthopaedics**	1	4	1	1	1	3	-	-	-	-	-	-
• **Extra-oral traction**	1	4		1			-	-	-	-	-	-
• **Arch lengthening & expansion**	1	4		1			-	-	-	-	-	-
• **Occlusion, oral physiology, malocclusions**	1	3			1		-	-	-	-	-	-
• **Orthodontic treatment; Phase I (levelling and alignment)**	1	3	1	1			-	-	-	-	-	-
• **Disturbances in dental development including impacted teeth**	1	3					-	-	-	-	-	-
• **Smile aesthetics**	1	3		1	1		-	-	-	-	-	-
• **Implants**	1	3					-	-	-	-	-	-
• **Teaching & learning**	-	3		1			-	-	-	-	-	-
Skills (S)												
• **Comprehensive Orthodontics**	-	-	-	-	-	-	-	-	-	-	-	6
• **Bonding**	-	-	-	-	-	-	-	-	-	-	1	-
• **Orthodontic Diagnostic & Treatment Planning skills**	-	-	1	-	-	-	-	-	6	-	-	-

Areas to be covered in this Module	SAQ	MCQ	TOACS	OOT (PAL)	OOT (Presentation)	OOT (JCM)	OOT (Lec/ Demo)	CL	CbD	Mini-CEX	DOPS	PPP
• Functional appliance (Removable)	-	-	-	-	-	-	-	1	-	-	1	
• Forsus appliance	-	-	-	-	-	-	-	1	-	-		-
• Expansion appliances	-	-	1	-	-	-	-	1	-	-	-	-
• Bite plates (ant/post), Erverdi Plate, Inclined planes	-	-	-	-	-	-	-	1	-	-	-	-
• Head gear, Face mask, Chin cup	-	-	1	-	-	-	-	1	-	-	-	-
• Implant placement	-	-	1	-	-	-	-	-	-	-	1	-
• Comprehensive case records	-	-	-	-	-	-	-	1	-	3	-	-
• Teaching of final year BDS	-	-	-	-	-	-	1	-	-	-	-	-
Attitudes (A)												
• Explaining the procedure before hand • Taking consent from the patient • Privacy of the patient • Comfort & Confidentiality of the patient • Radiation Safety	-	-	-	-	-	-	-	-	-	3	3	-
Total	8	30	7	6	3	3	1	6	6	6	6	6

Module-III: Assessment Method

Formative + Summative

During Module by Work Place Based Assessment (WPBA)

Knowledge

1. OOT (PAL)______________6
2. OOT (Presentation)________3
3. OOT (JCM)______________3

Skills + Attitudes

4. OOT (Lec/Demo) _______1
5. CL___________________6
6. CbD__________________6
7. Mini-CEX______________6
8. DOPS_________________6
9. PPP___________________6
10. CIT___________________As & when Required

End of Module Examination

Knowledge

11. SAQs_________________8
12. MCQs________________30

Skills + Attitudes

13. TOACS________________7

Module-III: Checklist

Name of Resident: ______________________________

Months	Practical work	Date	Signature of Supervisor
1st Month	Comprehensive Case Records (Two)		
2nd Month	Hyrax		
	Quad helix		
	W-arch		
	Nitinol expander		
3rd Month	Impression & Bite registration for functional appliance		
	Articulation & fabrication of functional appliance		
4th Month	Headgear		
	Chin cup		
	Face mask		
5th Month	Forsus Appliance		
6th Month	Bite planes (ant/post)		
	Inclined plane		
	Erverdi plate		
	Research Article 1 accepted for publication/published		

Chapter 11

MODULE-IV

LEARNING OBJECTIVES

By the end of the module, the trainee should be able to;

- Relate the current orthodontic appliances with the historic ones.
- Choose appropriate mechanics to carry out phase II & III of orthodontic treatment keeping in view the adult and adjunctive orthodontics and its impact on dentition, periodontium & TMJ
- Teach the subject of orthodontics & give demonstrations to final year BDS.
- Apply the knowledge of relapse for stability of attained orthodontic results.
- Undertake research work for dissertation writing.
- Demonstrate ability to take basic diagnostic records and interpretation and application of fixed orthodontic appliances
- Practice Kesling setup and fabricate various retention appliances.
- Analyse data for bio statistical use in research work.
- Demonstrate ability to counsel patient, obtain consent and preserve patient privacy and confidentiality.

Module-IV: Topics to be Covered

Knowledge			Skills and Attitudes			
Knowledge (K)	**Instructional Strategies (K)**	**Assessment Items (K)**	**Skills (S)**	**Attitudes (A)**	**Instructional Strategies (S & A)**	**Assessment Items (S & A)**

• History of orthodontics
• Appliance systems (Begg, Tip edge, Tweed, Damon, MBT, etc.)
• Orthodontic treatment Phase II
  • Overbite correction
  • Over jet correction
  • Closure of residual spaces
• Orthodontic treatment Phase III (finishing)
• TMJ, Adult orthodontics
• Adjunctive orthodontics
• Orthodontic research for dissertation writing
• Biostatistics
• Extraction vs non-extraction
• Periodontal problems
• Iatrogenic effects of orthodontic treatment
• Retention & relapse
• Teaching & learning
• Medical Writing
	• Self-study
	• Peer Assisted Learning (PAL) {lectures by third year residents}
	• Weekly presentation
	• Weekly journal club meeting (JCM)
		• End of module exam comprising of MCQs, SAQs & Viva
		• OOT (PAL)
		• OOT (Presentation)
		• OOT (JCM)
			• Comprehensive orthodontics
			• Orthodontic Diagnostic & Treatment planning
			• Piggy back arches
			• Segmental wire work
			• Kesling set up
			• Fixed wire work
			  • Arch forms
			  • 1st, 2nd, 3rd order bends
			  • Loops and springs
			  • Auxiliaries
			• Retainers
			  • Essex type
			  • Lingual
			  • Clip-on type
			• Analysis of biostatistics in research paper
			• Demonstrations & teaching of final year BDS
			• Comprehensive case record
			• Medical writing
				• Explaining the procedure before hand
				• Obtain patient's consent
				• Ensure Patient's comfort
				• Maintain privacy of the patient
				• Preserve Confidentiality of the patient
				• Radiation Safety
				• Recognise & inform the patient about oral health care
					• Peer Assisted Learning (PAL) (demonstrati ons by senior residents)
					• Self-practice
						• CbD
						• CL
						• DOPS
						• Mini-CEX
						• OOT (Lec/Demo)
						• PPP
						• TOACS
						• CIT
						• Acceptance of Research paper 1 for publication
						• Submission of synopsis for Dissertation

Module-IV: Reading List

	Topic	References
1	**History of orthodontics Appliance systems (Begg, Tip edge, Tweed, Damon, MBT, etc.),**	• Orthodontic treatment mechanics and preadjusted appliances, • Orthodontics Current Principles and Techniques, 6th Edition- Lee W Grabber, Robert L. Vanarsdall Jr Chapter15: Standard Edgewise: Tweed-Merrifield Philosophy, • Diagnosis, Treatment Planning, Milton B. Asbell, DDS, MSc, MA Cherry Hill, N. J., • AJODO. September 1990□A brief history of orthodontics, A brief history of orthodontics Milton B. Asbell, MA Cherry Hill, N. J • AJODO August 1990 • Volume 98 • Number 2, p 176-183
2	**Orthodontic treatment Phase II**	• Contemporary Orthodontics. 5th edition. William R Proffit, Henry W Fields, David M Sarver Chapter#15 The Second Stage of Comprehensive Treatment: Correction of Molar Relationship and Space Closure • Orthodontics Current Principles and Techniques, 6th Edition- Lee W Grabber, Robert L. Vanarsdall Jr chapter #17 Contemporary Straight Wire Biomechanics,
3	**Overbite correction**	• Contemporary Orthodontics. 5th edition. William R Proffit, Henry W Fields, David M Sarver chapter # 16 The Third Stage of Comprehensive Treatment: Finishing • Orthodontics Current Principles and Techniques, 6th Edition- Lee W Grabber, Robert L. Vanarsdall Jr chapter #16 Contemporary Treatment • Mechanics Using the Straight Wire Appliance
4	**Over jet correction**	• Contemporary Orthodontics. 5th edition. William R Proffit, Henry W Fields, David M Sarver chapter # 16 The Third Stage of Comprehensive Treatment: Finishing, • Orthodontics Current Principles and Techniques, 6th Edition- Lee W Grabber, Robert L. Vanarsdall Jr chapter #16 Contemporary Treatment • Mechanics Using the Straight Wire Appliance
5	**Closure of Residual spaces**	• Contemporary Orthodontics. 5th edition. William R Proffit, Henry W Fields, David M Sarver chapter # 16 Third Stage of Comprehensive Treatment: • Finishing, • Orthodontics Current Principles and Techniques, 6th Edition- Lee W Grabber, Robert L. Vanarsdall Jr chapter #16 Contemporary Treatment Mechanics Using the Straight Wire Appliance

Module-IV: Reading List (Continued)

	Topic	References
6	**Orthodontic treatment Phase III (finishing)**	• Contemporary Orthodontics. 5th edition. William R Proffit, Henry W Fields, David M Sarver chapter # 16 Third Stage of Comprehensive Treatment: Finishing • Orthodontics Current Principles and Techniques, 6th Edition- Lee W Grabber, Robert L. Vanarsdall Jr chapter #16 Contemporary Treatment Mechanics Using the Straight Wire Appliance
7	**TMJ**	• Orthodontics Current Principles and Techniques, 6th Edition- Lee W Grabber, Robert L. Vanarsdall Jr Chapter #13 Orthodontic Therapy and the Patient with Temporomandibular Disorder, • Mosby Orthodontic Review chapter #22 temporomandibular disorders: page#260, • Jaffery P OKeson Management of Temporomandibular Disorders and Occlusion, 6th Edition
8	**Adult orthodontics**	• Orthodontics Current Principles and Techniques, 6th Edition- Lee W Grabber, Robert L. Vanarsdall Jr chapter #24 Adult Interdisciplinary Therapy: Diagnosis and Treatment • Contemporary Orthodontics. 5th edition. William R Proffit, Henry W Fields, David M Sarver Chapter #18 Special Considerations in Treatment for Adults • Mosby Orthodontic Review: Chapter #17 Adult interdisciplinary orthodontic treatment
9	**Journals**	• AJODO, Seminars in Orthodontics, Angles Orthodontist, European Journal of orthodontics, Cochrane Reviews, Classical Articles

Module-IV: Table of Specifications

Areas to be covered in this Module	SAQ	MCQ	TOACS	OOT (PAL)	OOT (presentation)	OOT (JCM)	OOT (Lec/ Demo)	CL	CbD	Mini-CEX	DOPS	PPP
Knowledge (K)												
• History of orthodontics & Appliance systems	1	3	1	1	1							
• Orthodontic treatment Phase II & III		3										
• TMJ	1	3		1								
• Adult orthodontics		3		1	1							
• Adjunctive orthodontics	1	3										
• Periodontal problems related to appliance wear		3	1	1		3	-	-	-	-	-	-
• Extraction vs. non-extraction	1	3			1							
• Iatrogenic effects of orthodontic treatment		3		1								
• Retention & relapse		3										
• Research Methodology & Biostatistics	1	3		1								
Skills (S)												
• Comprehensive Orthodontics	-	-	-	-	-	-	-	-	-	-	-	6
• Arch wire selection and insertion	-	-	-	-	-	-	-	-	-	-	1	-
• Orthodontic Diagnostic & Treatment Planning skills	-	-	2	-	-	-	-	-	6	-	-	-
• Piggy back arches	-	-	-	-	-	-	-	-	-	-	1	-
• Segmental canine retraction	-	-	1	-	-	-	-	-	-	-	1	-
• Kesling set up	-	-	-	-	-	-	-	1	-	-	-	-

Module-IV: Table of Specifications (Continued)

Areas to be covered in this Module	SAQ	MCQ	TOACS	OOT (PAL)	OOT (presentation)	OOT (JCM)	OOT (Lec/ Demo)	CL	CbD	Mini-CEX	DOPS	PPP
• Fixed wire work	-	-	1	-	-	-	-	1	-	-	-	-
• Retainers	-	-	-	-	-	-	-	1	-	-	-	-
• Comprehensive case records	-	-	-	-	-	-	-	2	-	3	-	-
• Teaching of final year BDS	-	-	-	-	-	-	1	-	-	-	-	-
• Submission of Synopsis for Dissertation/Thesis	-	-	-	-	-	-	-	1	-	-	-	-
• Acceptance of research paper 1 for publication	-	-	-	-	-	-	-	1	-	-	-	-
Attitudes (A)												
• Explaining the procedure before hand • Taking consent from the patient • Privacy of the patient • Comfort of the patient • Confidentiality of the patient • Radiation Safety	-	-	-	-	-	-	-	-	-	3	3	-
Total	5	30	6	6	3	3	1	7	6	6	6	6

Module-IV: Assessment Method

Formative/Summative

During Module by Work Place Based Assessment (WPBA)

Knowledge

1. OOT (PAL)______________6
2. OOT (Presentation)_______3
3. OOT (JCM)______________3

Skills + Attitudes

4. OOT (Lec/Demo)_______1
5. CL___________________7
6. CbD__________________6
7. Mini-CEX______________6
8. DOPS_________________6
9. PPP__________________6
10. CIT__________________As & when Required

End of Module Examination

Knowledge

11. SAQs_________________5
12. MCQs________________30

Skills & Attitudes

13. TOACS_______________6

Module-IV: Checklist

Name of Resident: ____________________________

Months	Practical work	Date	Signature of Supervisor
1st Month	Comprehensive Case Record (Two)		
2nd Month	*Loops;* T, opus, reverse helical, bull, Lolly pop		
	Mulligan Mechanics: out bend, in bend, toe in, toe out, anchor bend		
3rd Month	Arch forms		
	1st, 2nd, 3rd order bends,		
4th Month	*Intrusion arches:* Utility arch, Burstone Arch *Auxiliaries:* Rotating springs, Torqueing springs		
5th Month	Kesling setup		
	Acceptance of Research paper 1 for publication		
6th Month	Approval of synopsis for Dissertation/Thesis		
	Retainers Essex type, Fixed retainer Clip on retainer		

Chapter 12

Intermediate Exam (At the Completion of Modules I-IV)

Summative Assessment

		Module I	Module II	Module III	Module IV	Total
Knowledge						
1.	SAQs	2	2	3	3	10
2.	MCQs	30	30	30	30	120
Skills + Attitudes						
3.	TOACS (12 Stations as per TOS)	3	3	3	3	12

Chapter 13

MODULE-V

LEARNING OBJECTIVES

By the end of the module, the trainee should be able to;

- Plan and execute orthognathic surgical cases with reference to facial asymmetries, Cleft Lip & Palate and skeletal disharmonies.
- Solve problems related to high frenal attachment and severe tooth rotations.
- Teach the subject of orthodontics & give demonstrations to final year BDS.
- Undertake a research project leading to publication & submission of synopsis for research paper 1.
- Take basic diagnostic record, interpret it and carry out fixed orthodontic treatment using various mechanics.
- Demonstrate ability to counsel patient, obtain consent and preserve patient privacy and confidentiality

Module-V: Topics to be Covered

Knowledge			Skills and Attitudes			
Knowledge (K)	**Instructional Strategies (K)**	**Assessment Items (K)**	**Skills (S)**	**Attitudes (A)**	**Instructional Strategies (S&A)**	**Assessment Items (S&A)**
• Minor Oral surgery (CSF, high frenum, etc.) • Facial asymmetries • Orthognathic surgery • Cleft Lip & Palate • Systemic effects of orthodontic treatment • Trauma and orthodontics • Orthodontic research	• Self-study • Peer Assisted Learning (PAL) {lectures by fourth year residents} • Weekly presentation • Weekly journal club meeting (JCM)	• End of module exam comprising of MCQs, SAQs & Viva • OOT (PAL) • OOT (Presentati on) • OOT (JCM)	• CSF procedure • Comprehensive orthodontics • Orthodontic Diagnostic & Treatment planning skills • Prediction tracing • Face bow record and mounting • Model surgery • Splint fabrication & insertion • Demonstrations & teaching of final year BDS	• Explaining the procedure before hand • Obtain patient's consent • Ensure Patient's comfort • Maintain privacy of the patient • Preserve Confidentiality of the patient • Radiation safety	• Peer Assisted Learning (PAL) (demonstrati ons by senior residents) • Self-practice	• CbD • CL • DOPS • OOT (Lecture/Dem o) • PPP • TOACS • CIT

Module-V: Reading List

	Topic	References
1	**Minor Oral surgery (CSF, high frenum, etc.)**	• Contemporary Orthodontics. 5th edition. William R Proffit, Henry W Fields, David M Sarver: Chapter 16 • Orthodontics Current Principles and Techniques, 6th Edition- Lee W Grabber, Robert L. Vanarsdall Jr: Chapter 23
2	**Facial asymmetries**	• Contemporary Orthodontics. 5th edition. William R Proffit, Henry W Fields, David M Sarver: Chapter 13 & 19 • Orthodontics Current Principles and Techniques, 6th Edition- Lee W Grabber, Robert L. Vanarsdall Jr: Chapter 25 • Contemporary treatment of dentofacial deformity: Chapter 17
3	**Orthognathic Surgery**	• Contemporary Orthodontics. 5th edition. William R Proffit, Henry W Fields, David M Sarver: Chapter 19 • Orthodontics Current Principles and Techniques, 6th Edition- Lee W Grabber, Robert L. Vanarsdall Jr: Chapter 25 • Contemporary treatment of dentofacial deformity: Part III • Essentials of Orthognathic Surgery
4	**Cleft lip and palate**	• Contemporary Orthodontics. 5th edition. William R Proffit, Henry W Fields, David M Sarver: Chapter 7 • Orthodontics Current Principles and Techniques, 6th Edition- Lee W Grabber, Robert L. Vanarsdall Jr: Chapter 26
5	**Systemic effects of orthodontic treatment**	• Contemporary Orthodontics. 5th edition. William R Proffit, Henry W Fields, David M Sarver: Chapter 8 • Postgraduate Notes in Orthodontics, 5th Edition-Bristol: Chapter 11
6	**Trauma and orthodontics**	• Contemporary Orthodontics. 5th edition. William R Proffit, Henry W Fields, David M Sarver: Chapter 12 • Postgraduate Notes in Orthodontics, 5th Edition-Bristol: Chapter 11
7	**Comprehensive Orthodontics**	• Contemporary Orthodontics. 5th edition. William R Proffit, Henry W Fields, David M Sarver: Chapter 10, Chapter 14-17 • Orthodontics Current Principles and Techniques, 6th Edition- Lee W Grabber, Robert L. Vanarsdall Jr: Chapter 16
8	**Orthodontic diagnostic and treatment planning**	• Contemporary Orthodontics. 5th edition. William R Proffit, Henry W Fields, David M Sarver: Chapter 6, 7 • Orthodontics Current Principles and Techniques, 6th Edition- Lee W Grabber, Robert L. Vanarsdall Jr: Chapter 13
9	**Prediction tracing**	• Facial and dental planning for orthodontists: chapter 7 • Essentials of Orthognathic surgery: Chapter 3 • Contemporary Treatment of Dentofacial Deformity. William R Proffit, Raymond P White, David M Sarver: Chapter 6
10	**Facebow record and mounting**	• The Recording and Transfer of Orthognathic Planning Data Mohammad Anwar Bamber and Edwin Payne
11	**Model Surgery**	• Contemporary Treatment of Dentofacial Deformity. William R Proffit, Raymond P White, David M Sarver: Chapter 6
12	**Splint fabrication and insertion**	• Management of temporomandibular disorders and occlusion Jaffery P Okeson: Chapter 15
13	**Journals**	• AJODO, Seminars in Orthodontics, Angles Orthodontist, European Journal of orthodontics, Cochrane Reviews, Classical Articles

Module-V: Table of Specifications

Areas to be covered in this Module	SAQ	MCQ	TOACS	OOT (PAL)	OOT (presentation)	OOT (JCM)	OOT (Lecture/ Demo)	CL	CbD	DOPS	PPP
Knowledge (K)											
• Minor Oral surgery (CSF, high frenum, etc.)	1	3	1	1	1	-	-	-	-	-	-
• Facial asymmetries	1	6		1		-	-	-	-	-	-
• Orthognathic surgery	1	6		1	1	3	-	-	-	-	-
• Cleft Lip & Palate	1	6	1	1		-	-	-	-	-	-
• Systemic effects of orthodontic treatment	1	6		1	1	-	-	-	-	-	-
• Trauma and orthodontics		3		1		-	-	-	-	-	-
Skills (S)											
• Comprehensive Orthodontics	-	-	-	-	-	-	-	-	-	-	6
• Anterior Retraction (Helices with Power O/class II Mechanics	-	-	-	-	-	-	-	-	-	1	-
• CSF procedure/Frenectomy/Gingivectomy/ gingivoplasty	-	-	-	-	-	-	-	-	-	1	-
• Orthodontic Diagnostic & Treatment Planning skills	-	-	1	-	-	-	-	-	6	-	-
• Prediction tracing	-	-	1	-	-	-	-	1	-	-	-
• Face bow record and mounting	-	-	1	-	-	-	-	1	-	1	-
• Model surgery	-	-	1	-	-	-	-	1	-	-	-
• Splint fabrication	-	-	1	-	-	-	-	3	-	-	-
• Demonstrations & teaching of final year BDS	-	-		-	-	-	1		-	-	-

Areas to be covered in this Module	SAQ	MCQ	TOACS	OOT (PAL)	OOT (presentation)	OOT (JCM)	OOT (Lecture/ Demo)	CL	CbD	DOPS	PPP
Attitudes (A)											
• **Explaining the procedure before hand** • **Taking consent from patient** • **Informed consent** • **Privacy of patient** • **Comfort of patient** • **Confidentiality of patient** • **Radiation Safety**	-	-	-	-	-	-	-	-	-	3	-
Total	5	30	7	6	3	3	1	6	6	6	6

Module-V: Assessment Method

Formative + Summative Assessment

During Module by Work Place Based Assessment (WPBA)

Knowledge

1. OOT (PAL)______________6
2. OOT (Presentation)_______3
3. OOT (JCM)______________3

Skills + Attitudes

4. OOT (Lec/Demo)_______1
5. CL____________________6
6. CbD__________________6
7. DOPS_________________6
8. PPP__________________6
9. CIT____________________As & when Required

End of Module Examination

Knowledge

10. SAQs_________________5
11. MCQs_________________30

Skill + Attitudes

12. TOACS________________7

Module-V: Checklist

Name of Resident: ______________________________

Months	Practical work	Date	Signature of Supervisor
1st Month	Prediction tracing		
2nd Month	Face bow Record and Mounting		
3rd Month	Model surgery		
4th Month	Surgical Splint fabrication (Intermediate+ Final)		
5th Month	Stabilization Appliance		
6th Month	Anterior positioning Appliance		
	Synopsis for research article 2 Approved by the supervisor		

Chapter 14

MODULE-VI

LEARNING OBJECTIVES

By the end of the module, the trainee should be able to;

- Identify and manage the cases of Distraction Osteogenesis, Obstructive Sleep Apnea and Lingual orthodontics.
- Describe the use of magnets in orthodontics.
- Teach the subject of orthodontics & give demonstrations to final year BDS.
- Undertake clinical audit.
- Develop and run specialist practice independently keeping in view the medicolegal aspects of health provision.
- Submit research work (paper 1) for publication.
- Take basic diagnostic record, interpret it and carry out fixed orthodontic treatment using distalizers and fixed functional appliances.
- Demonstrate ability to counsel patient, obtain consent and preserve patient privacy and confidentiality

Module-VI: Topics to be Covered

Knowledge			Skills and Attitudes			
Knowledge (K)	**Instructional Strategies (K)**	**Assessment Items (K)**	**Skills (S)**	**Attitudes (A)**	**Instructional Strategies (S & A)**	**Assessment Items (S & A)**

• Distraction Osteogenesis
• Obstructive sleep apnea
• Magnets
• Lingual orthodontics
• Clinical Audit
• Clinical Governance
• Medicolegal aspects of practice
• Medical writing
	• Self-study
	• Peer Assisted Learning (PAL) {lectures by fourth year residents}
	• Weekly presentation
	• Weekly journal club meeting (JCM
		• End of module exam comprising of MCQs, SAQs & Viva
		• OOT (PAL)
		• OOT (Presentation)
		• OOT (JCM)
			• Comprehensive orthodontics
			• Orthodontic Diagnostic & Treatment planning skills
			• Crimpable hook
			• Ball stop
			• Pendulum appliance
			• Distal jet
			• Jones jig
			• Fixed functional appliances;
			  • Mara
			  • Sabbagh universal spring
			  • Bite corrector
			  • Jasper jumper, etc.
			• Demonstrations & teaching of final year BDS
			• Comprehensive case records (Debonding)
			• Synopsis writing for Research Paper 2
				• Explaining the procedure before hand
				• Obtain patient's consent
				• Ensure patient's comfort
				• Maintain privacy of the patient
				• Preserve Confidentiality of the patient
				• Radiation safety
					• Peer Assisted Learning (PAL) (demonstrations by senior residents)
					• Self-practice
						• CbD
						• CL
						• DOPS
						• Mini-CEX
						• OOT (Lec/Demo)
						• PPP
						• TOACS
						• CIT
						• Submission of synopsis for research paper 2

Module-VI: Reading List

	Topic	References
1	**Distraction osteogenesis**	• Contemporary Treatment of Dentofacial Deformity. William R Proffit, Raymond P White, David M Sarver Chapter number 12, page 357 • "Craniofacial Distraction Osteogenesis" by Mikhail L. Samchukov. • "Orthodontics. Current principles and techniques by Graber. 5th edition, Chapter number 25, Page 1053 • Seminar in Orthodontics, March 1999, Volume 5, Issue 1, p1-73, Distraction Osteogenesis.
2	**Obstructive sleep apnea**	• "Postgraduate notes in Orthodontics" by Bristol, 5th edition, page 241. • "Orthodontics. Current principles and techniques by Graber. 6th edition • Seminar in Orthodontics, June 2009, Volume 15, Issue 2, p85-158, Obstructive Sleep Apnea Syndrome: A Review and Dentofacial Implications.
3	**Magnets**	• Contemporary Orthodontics. 5th edition. William R Proffit, Henry W Fields, David M Sarver, pages 324 and 560. • Dentofacial Orthopaedics with Functional Appliances, T M Graber
4	**Lingual orthodontics**	• Contemporary Orthodontics by William R Proffit, pages 377, 667 and 670-671 • Seminars in Orthodontics, September 2006, Volume 12, Issues 3, p 151- 214, Lingual Orthodontics • Orthodontics Current Principles and Techniques, 5th Edition- Lee W Grabber, Robert L. Vanarsdall Jr, Chapter number 18
5	**Clinical audit, clinical governance**	• Postgraduate notes in Orthodontics" by Bristol, 5th edition, page 232-233.
6	**Medicolegal aspects of practice**	• Pharande SV, Potnis S, Jamenis S, Jamenis R. Legal Concerns for an Orthodontist. J Ind Orthod Soc 2012; 46(1):56-57.
		Skills
7	**Comprehensive orthodontics**	• Contemporary Orthodontics. 5th edition. William R Proffit, Henry W Fields, David M Sarver Chapter 10. • Orthodontics Current Principles and Techniques, 5th Edition- Lee W Grabber, Robert L. Vanarsdall Jr, Chapter number 16.
8	**Orthodontic diagnostic and treatment planning skills:**	• Participation in weekly treatment planning sessions every Thursday • Contemporary Orthodontics. 5th edition. William R Proffit, Henry W Fields, David M Sarver, Chapter 6 and Chapter 7. • Contemporary Treatment of Dentofacial Deformity. William R Proffit, Raymond P White, David M Sarver Chapter number 6 • Orthodontics Current Principles and Techniques, 5th Edition- Lee W Grabber, Robert L. Vanarsdall Jr Chapter number 2.

Module-VI: Reading List (Continued)

	Topic	References
9	**Crimpable hooks, ball stops**	Instruction manual PDF, Balls and Stops, www.americanortho.com
10	**Pendulum appliance**	• Orthodontics Current Principles and Techniques, 5th Edition- Lee W Grabber, Robert L. Vanarsdall Jr • Orthodontics Current Principles and Techniques, 4th Edition- Lee W Grabber, Robert L. Vanarsdall Jr Chapter number 12. • Contemporary Orthodontics. 5th edition. William R Proffit, Henry W Fields, David M Sarver
11	**Distal jet**	• Orthodontics Current Principles and Techniques, 4th Edition- Lee W Grabber, Robert L. Vanarsdall Jr Chapter number 12. • Instruction manual PDF. Distal Jet. American Orthodontics, www.americanortho.com
12	**Fixed functional appliances**	• Orthodontics Current Principles and Techniques, 4th Edition- Lee W Grabber, Robert L. Vanarsdall Jr, Chapter number 12., Functional Graber • Contemporary Orthodontics. 5th edition. William R Proffit, Henry W Fields, David M Sarver • MARA instruction manual PDF. www.aoaaccess.com • SABBAGH instruction manual PDF. https://www.dentaurum.de/eng/sus2-sabbagh-universal-spring-cd-rom
13	**Journals**	• AJODO, Seminars in Orthodontics, Angles Orthodontist, European Journal of orthodontics, Cochrane Reviews, Classical Articles

Module-VI: Table of Specifications

Areas to be covered in this Module	SAQ	MCQ	TOACS	OOT (PAL)	OOT (Presentation)	OOT (JCM)	OOT (Lec/Demo)	CL	CbD	DOPS	PPP
Knowledge (K)											
• Distraction osteogenesis	1	6	1	1	1						
• Obstructive sleep apnea	1	6		1							
• Magnets	-	3		1	1						
• Lingual orthodontics	1	6	1	1		3	-	-	-	-	-
• Clinical audit, Clinical governance	1	6		1	1						
• Medicolegal aspects of practice	1	3		1							
Skills (S)											
• Comprehensive Orthodontics	-	-	1	-	-	-	-		-	-	6
• Anterior Retraction with Loops	-	-	-	-	-	-	-	-	-	1	-
• Orthodontic Diagnostic & Treatment Planning skills	-	-	-	-	-	-	-	-	6	-	-
• Crimpable hook, Ball stop	-	-	-	-	-	-	-	-	-	1	-
• Pendulum appliance	-	-	1	-	-	-	-	1	-	-	
• Distal jet	-	-		-	-	-	-	1	-	1	-
• Jones jig	-	-		-	-	-	-	1	-		
• Fixed functional appliances; • Mara • Sabbagh universal spring • Bite corrector • Jasper jumper, etc.	-	-	1	-	-	-	-	1 1 1 1		-	-

Module-VI: Table of Specifications (Continued)

Areas to be covered in this Module	SAQ	MCQ	TOACS	OOT (PAL)	OOT (Presentation)	OOT (JCM)	OOT (Lec/Demo)	CL	CbD	DOPS	PPP
• Demonstrations & teaching of final year BDS											
• Comprehensive orthodontic case record (Debonded case)	-	-	-	-	-	-	-	1	-	-	-
Submission of synopsis for research paper 2	-	-	-	-	-	-	-	1	-	-	-
Attitudes (A)											
• Explaining the procedure before hand • Taking consent from patient • Informed consent • Privacy of patient • Comfort of patient • Confidentiality of patient • Radiation Safety		-	-	-	-	-	-	-	-	3	-
Total	5	30	5	6	3	3	1	9	6	6	6

Module VI: Assessment Method

Formative + Summative Assessment

During Module by Work Place Based Assessment (WPBA)

Knowledge

1. OOT (PAL)______________6
2. OOT (Presentation)_______3
3. OOT (JCM)______________3

Skills + Attitudes

4. OOT (Lec/Demo)_______1
5. CL____________________9
6. CbD___________________6
7. DOPS__________________6
8. PPP___________________6
9. CIT____________________As & when Required

End of Module Examination

Knowledge

10. SAQs_________________5
11. MCQs________________30

Skills & Attitudes

12. TOACS________________5

Module-VI: Checklist

Name of Resident: ______________________________

Months	Practical work	Date	Signature of Supervisor
1st Month	Comprehensive case record of debonded cases & ABO Grading		
	Ball stop		
2nd Month	Pendulum Appliance		
3rd Month	Distal Jet		
	Wilson Arch		
4th Month	MARA		
	Sabbagh Universal Spring		
5th Month	Jones Jig		
6th Month	Bite Corrector		
	Jasper Jumper		

Chapter 15

MODULE-VII

LEARNING OBJECTIVES

By the end of the module, the trainee should be able to;

- Apply the knowledge of indirect bonding, self-ligating brackets and LASERS in clinical orthodontics.
- Teach the subject of orthodontics & give demonstrations to final year BDS.
- Undertake a research project leading to publication & submission of synopsis for research paper 2.
- Use Dolphin imaging and digitized landmark identification for cephalometric analysis and Visual Treatment Objective (VTO).
- Demonstrate ability to counsel patient, obtain consent and preserve patient privacy and confidentiality

Module-VII: Topics to be Covered

Knowledge			Skills and Attitudes			
Knowledge (K)	**Instructional Strategies (K)**	**Assessment Items (K)**	**Skills (S)**	**Attitudes (A)**	**Instructional Strategies (S & A)**	**Assessment Items (S & A)**
• Indirect bonding • Self-ligating brackets • LASERS • Aligners	• Self-study • Peer Assisted Learning (PAL) {Registrar/Senior registrar} • Weekly presentation • Weekly journal club meeting (JCM)	• End of module exam comprising of MCQs, SAQs & Viva • OOT (PAL) • OOT (Presentation) • OOT (JCM)	• Comprehensive Orthodontics • Orthodontic Diagnostic & Treatment planning • Aligners • Indirect bonding • Dolphin imaging • Digitized landmark identification & ceph analysis • Demonstrations & teaching of final year BDS • Undertaking a research project leading to publication (synopsis for paper 2) • Comprehensive case records (Debonding)	• Explaining the procedure before hand • Obtain patient's consent • Ensure Patient's comfort • Maintain privacy of the patient • Preserve Confidentiality of the patient • Radiation safety	• Peer Assisted Learning (PAL) (demonstrations by Registrar/ Senior Registrar) • Self-practice	• CbD • CL • DOPS • Mini-CEX • OOT (Lecture/ Demo) • PPP • TOACS • CIT • LCC • SCCs • Acceptance of Research paper 2 for publication • Dissertation Submission

Module-VII: Reading List

	Topic	References
1	**Indirect bonding**	• Seminars in Orthodontics, March 2007, Volume 13, Issue 1(Indirect Precision Bonding) • Bonding in Orthodontics, Chapter 27, Orthodontics Current Principles and Techniques, 6th Edition- Lee W Grabber, Robert L. Vanarsdall Jr
2	**Self-ligating brackets**	• Self-ligating brackets, chapter 17, Orthodontics Current Principles and Techniques, 6th Edition- Lee W Grabber, Robert L. Vanarsdall Jr • Seminars in Orthodontics, March 2008, Volume 14, Issue 1
3	**Lasers**	• Lasers in Orthodontics, Chapter 30, Orthodontics Current Principles and Techniques, 6th Edition- Lee W Grabber, Robert L. Vanarsdall Jr
4	**Aligners**	• Clear Aligners, Chapter 19, Orthodontics Current Principles and Techniques, 6th Edition- Lee W Grabber, Robert L. Vanarsdall Jr • A perspective in accelerated orthodontics with aligner treatment. Seminars in Orthodontics, Published online: November 8, 2016 • Improving the predictability of clear aligners. Steven Jay Bowman. Seminars in Orthodontics. Published online: October 17, 2016 • Orthodontic clear aligner treatment. Timothy T. Wheeler. Seminars in Orthodontics. Published online: October 17, 2016
5	**Journals**	• AJODO • Seminars in Orthodontics • Angles Orthodontist • European Journal of orthodontics • Cochrane Reviews • Classical Articles

Module-VII: Table of Specifications

Areas to be covered in this Module	SAQ	MCQ	TOACS	OOT (PAL)	OOT (Presentation)	OOT (JCM)	OOT (Lecture/ Demo)	CL	CbD	DOPS	LCC	SCCs	PPP
Knowledge (K)													
• Indirect bonding	1	8	1	1	1	3							
• Self-ligating brackets	2	8		1			-	-	-	-	-	-	-
• LASERS	1	7	1	1	1								
• Aligners	1	7		1	1								
Skills (S)													
• Comprehensive Orthodontics	-	-	-	-	-	-	-	-	-	-	-	-	6
• Finishing and detailing	-	-	-	-	-	-	-	-	-	1	-	-	-
• Orthodontic Diagnostic & Treatment Planning skills	-	-	1	-	-	-	-	-	6	-	1	5	-
• Indirect bonding	-	-	-	-	-	-	-	-	-	1	-	-	-
• Dolphin imaging	-	-	1	-	-	-	-	1	-	-	-	-	-
• Digitized landmark identification & ceph analysis e.g., view box	-	-	1	-	-	-	-	2	-	-	-	-	-
• Demonstrations & teaching of final year BDS	-	-	-	-	-	-	1	-	-	-	-	-	-
• Comprehensive case records (Debonded case)	-	-	-	-	-	-	-	1	-	-	-	-	-
• Explaining the procedure before hand • Taking consent from patient • Informed consent • Privacy of patient • Comfort of patient • Confidentiality of patient • Radiation Safety	-	-	-	-	-	-	-	-	-	2	-	-	-
Total	5	30	5	4	3	3	1	4	6	4	1	5	6

Module-VII: Assessment Method

Formative/Summative Assessment

During Module by Work Place Based Assessment (WPBA)

Knowledge

1. OOT (PAL)______________4
2. OOT (Presentation)________3
3. OOT (JCM)______________3

Skills + Attitudes

4. OCT (Lec/Demo)_______1
5. CL____________________4
6. CbD__________________6
7. DOPS_________________4
8. PPP___________________6
9. CIT___________________As & when Required

EOM Examination Knowledge

10. SAQs_________________5
11. MCQs________________30

Skills + Attitudes

12. TOACS_______________5
13. LCC__________________1
14. SCCs_________________5

Module-VII: Checklist

Name of Resident: ______________________________

Months	Practical work	Date	Signature of Supervisor
1st Month	Comprehensive case record of debonded cases+ ABO Grading		
2nd Month	Digitized landmarks identification & Cephalometric Analysis e.g., View box		
3rdMonth	Dolphin imaging 1		
4th Month	Dolphin imaging 2		
5th Month	Indirect bonding		
6th Month	Research Article 2 accepted for publication/published		

Chapter 16

MODULE-VIII

LEARNING OBJECTIVES

By the end of the module, the trainee should be able to;

- Impart leadership skill through staff management; patient and financial record keeping; observing disciplinary action; and, store keeping.
- Teach the subject of orthodontics & give demonstrations to final year BDS.
- Submit research work (paper 2) for publication.
- Solve past papers and MCQs.
- Analyse critically the articles of journals.
- Comply with the welfare & rights of staff members, confidentiality of patients' record and honesty.

Module-VIII: Topics to be Covered

Knowledge			Skills and Attitudes			
Knowledge (K)	**Instructional Strategies (K)**	**Assessment Items (K)**	**Skills (S)**	**Attitudes (A)**	**Instructional Strategies (S &A)**	**Assessment Items (S & A)**
• Management of staff • Disciplinary procedures • Patients' record keeping • Financial record keeping • Store keeping • Past FCPS papers • MCQs • Journals • Medical writing	• Self-study • Peer Assisted Learning (PAL) {Registrar/ Senior registrar} • Weekly presentation • Weekly journal club meeting (JCM)	• End of module exam comprising of MCQs, SAQs & Viva • OOT (PAL) • OOT (Presentation) • OOT (JCM)	• Comprehensive Orthodontics • Orthodontic Diagnostic & Treatment planning • Staff management • Disciplinary procedures • Patients' record keeping • Financial record keeping • Store keeping • Demonstrations & teaching of final year BDS • Comprehensive case records (Debonding) • Medical writing	• Consider the rights and welfare of staff members • Maintain confidentiality of patients' record • Exhibit honesty	• Peer Assisted Learning (PAL) (demonstration by Registrar/ • Senior Registrar) • Self-practice	• CbD • CL • DOPS • Mini-CEX • PPP • TOACS • CIT • LCC • SCCs • Dissertation Approval

Module-VIII: Reading List

	Topic	References
1	**Management of staff** **Patients' record keeping** **Financial record keeping** **Store keeping** **Disciplinary procedures**	• Financial Management: Theory & Practice by Eugene F. Brigham • Seminars 2016 on Management & Leadership
2	**Journals**	• AJODO • Angles Orthodontist • European Journal of orthodontics • Cochrane Reviews • Classical Articles • Seminars
3	**Medical writing**	• A to Z of Medical writing by Tim Albert • Scientific writing Jennifer Peat
4	**MCQs and SAQs Writing**	• MCQs and SAQs Writing guidelines by CPSP

Module-VIII: Table of Specifications

Areas to be covered in this Module	SAQ	MCQ	TOACS	OOT (PAL)	OOT (presentation)	OOT (JCM)	OOT (Lecture /Demo)	CL	CbD	DOPS	LCC	SCCs	PPP
Knowledge (K)													
• Management of staff	1	6	1	1	1								
• Disciplinary procedures	1	6		1									
• Patients' record keeping	1	6		1	1								
• Financial record keeping	1	6		1		3	-	-	-	-	-	-	-
• Store keeping	1	6	1	1	1								
• Journals	-	-	-	-	-								
Skills (S)													
• Comprehensive Orthodontics	-	-	-	-	-	-	-	-	-	-	-	-	6
• Debonding & Retention	-	-	-	-	-	-	-	-	-	-	-	-	-
• Orthodontic Diagnostic & Treatment Planning	-	-	2	-	-	-	-	-	-	1	1	5	-
• Staff management	-	-	-	-	-	-	-	-	6				-
• Disciplinary procedures	-	-	-	-	-	-	-	1	-	-	-	-	-
• Patients' record keeping	-	-	-	-	-	-	-	-	-	1	-	-	-
• Financial record keeping	-	-	-	-	-	-	-	1	-	-	-	-	-
• Store keeping	-	-	-	-	-	-	-	1	-	-	-	-	-
• Demonstrations & teaching of final year	-	-	-	-	-	-	-	1	-	-	-	-	-
• Comprehensive case records (Debonding)	-	-	-	-	-	-	1	-	-	-	-	-	-

Module-VIII: Table of Specifications (Continued)

Areas to be covered in this Module	SAQ	MCQ	TOACS	OOT (PAL)	OOT (presentation)	OOT (JCM)	OOT (Lecture /Demo)	CL	CbD	DOPS	LCC	SCCs	PPP
• Acceptance of Research paper 2 for publication	-	-	-	-	-	-	-	-	-	-	-	-	-
• Submission of Dissertation/Thesis	-	-	-	-	-	-	-	1	-	-	-	-	-
Attitudes (A)													
• Considerations about the rights of staff • Welfare of staff • Confidentiality of patients' record • Honesty	-	-	-	-	-	-	-	-	-	2	-	-	-
Total	5	30	4	5	3	3	1	5	6	4	1	5	6

Module VIII: Assessment Method

Formative/Summative Assessment

During Module by Work Place Based Assessment (WPBA)

Knowledge

1. OOT (PAL)_____________5
2. OOT (Presentation)_______3
3. OOT (JCM)_____________3

Skills + Attitudes

4. OOT (Lec/Demo)_______1
5. CL__________________5
6. CbD_________________6
7. DOPS________________4
8. PPP_________________6
9. CIT__________________As & when Required

End of Module Examination

Knowledge

10. SAQs________________5
11. MCQs_______________30

Skills & Attitudes

12. TOACS_______________4
13. LCC_________________1
14. SCCs________________5

Module-VIII: Checklist

Name of Resident: ____________________________

Months	Practical work	Date	Signature of Supervisor
1st Month	Comprehensive case records of debonded cases+ ABO Grading		
2nd Month	Financial record keeping		
3rd Month	Store keeping		
4th Month	Staff management		
5th Month	Patients' record keeping		
6th Month	Acceptance/approval of Dissertation/Thesis		

Chapter 17

EXIT EXAM (AT THE COMPLETION OF MODULES I-VIII)

SUMMATIVE ASSESSMENT

	Module I	Module II	Module III	Module IV	Module V	Module VI	Module VII	Module VIII	Total
Knowledge									
SAQs	1	1	1	2	1	1	1	2	10
MCQs	15	15	15	15	15	15	15	15	120
Skills + Attitudes									
TOACS (12 Stations as per TOS)	1	1	1	2	1	1	1	2	12
Long Clinical Case									1
SCCs 1-5 (Trainees' own treated cases)									
Case 1. Surgical/Multidisciplinary/CLP									1
Case 2. Growth Modification									1
Case 3. Comprehensive Orthodontics									1
Case 4. Comprehensive Orthodontics									1

Chapter 18

BI-ANNUAL REVIEW PROFORMA (B-ARP)

Name of Resident: ____________________________

Module: _________________________

Assessment Items	Knowledge					Skills								Attitudes		
	PAL	Presentation	JCM	EOM Exam MCQ SAQ	KNOWLEDGE TOTAL	CbD	PPP	DOPS	Mini-CEX	OOT	EOM Exam LCC, SCC, TOACS	SKILLS TOTAL	DOPS	Mini-CEX	OOT	ATTITUDES TOTAL
	% age of Marks Obtained					% age of Marks Obtained							% age of Marks Obtained			
Jan/July																
Feb/Aug																
March/Sep																
April/Oct																
May/Nov																
June/Dec																
Total of %ages																

Skills	
CL	**Synopsis/Dissertation/ Research Paper 1/ Research Paper 2**
Complete/Incomplete	
Jan/July	
Feb/Aug	
March/Sep	
April/Oct	
May/Nov	
June/Dec	
Total of %ages	

Promotion Criteria for Modules I, II, III, V, VI, VII

Preferred Promotion Criteria

Knowledge 60%	(Same Module) ☐
Skills 60%	(Same Module) ☐
Attitudes 60%	(Same Module) ☐
CL completed	(Same Module) ☐
Synopsis/Dissertation/Research paper 1/Research paper 2	(Same Module) ☐

Mandatory Promotion Criteria

Supplementary EOM exam passed	(previous Module) ☐
Reassessments passed	(previous Module) ☐
CL completed	(previous Module) ☐
Synopsis/Dissertation/Research paper 1/Research paper 2	(previous Module) ☐

For unconditional promotion to the next module it is must to meet both the preferred and mandatory promotion criteria. For promotion, the trainee has to fulfil at least the mandatory promotion criteria. If preferred promotion criteria are not fully met, the trainee will be conditionally promoted to the next module.

Promotion Criteria for Module IV, VIII
All of the above are mandatory

Remarks:____

Chapter 19

SAMPLE OF SCHEDULES

CbD/CL/PAL/PPP (6 per Module for each Resident)

	Jan	Feb	March	April	May	June
Resident 1	S-I	SR-I	SR-II	S-II	S-I	SR-I
Resident 2	S-II	S-I	SR-I	SR-I	S-II	SR-II
Resident 3	SR-I	S-II	S-I	SR-II	SR-I	S-I
Resident 4	SR-II	SR-I	S-II	S-I	SR-II	S-II
Resident 5	S-I	SR-II	SR-I	S-II	S-I	SR-I
Resident 6	S-II	S-I	SR-II	SR-I	S-II	SR-II
Resident 7	SR-I	S-II	S-I	SR-II	SR-I	S-II
Resident 8	SR-II	SR-I	S-II	S-I	SR-II	SR-I
Resident 9	S-I	SR-II	SR-I	S-II	S-I	SR-II
Resident 10	S-II	S-I	SR-II	SR	S-II	S-I

DOPS/Mini-CEX/Presentation/JCM (3 per Module for each Resident)

	Feb	April	June
Resident 1	S-I	SR-I	SR-II
Resident 2	S-II	S-I	SR-I
Resident 3	SR-I	S-II	S-I
Resident 4	SR-II	SR-I	S-II
Resident 5	S-I	SR-II	SR-I
Resident 6	S-II	S-I	SR-II
Resident 7	SR-I	S-II	S-I
Resident 8	SR-II	SR-I	S-II
Resident 9	S-I	SR-II	SR-I
Resident 10	S-II	S-I	SR-II

Observation of Teaching/ Demonstration (1 per Module for each Resident)

Resident 1	SR-I
Resident 2	SR-II
Resident 3	S-I
Resident 4	S-II
Resident 5	SR-I
Resident 6	SR-II
Resident 7	S-I
Resident 8	S-II
Resident 9	SR-I
Resident10	SR-II

S-I Supervisor I
S-II Supervisor II
SR-I Senior Registrar -I
SR-II Senior Registrar-II

Chapter 20

SAMPLE OF WEEKLY TIME TABLE

Day	TIME	ACTIVITY
Monday	0830 – 1000hrs 1000 – 1100hrs 1100 -1200hrs 1000-1400hrs	Journal Club and MCQs/SAQs Discussion Lecture for final year BDS & Residents Demo: Ceph/Wire work/Cast (BDS) Clinical Work
Tuesday	0830 – 1000hrs 1000- 1200hrs 1000-1400hrs	Orthodontic Presentation Demo: Ceph/Wire work/Cast (BDS) Clinical Work
Wednesday	0800 – 0900hrs 0900 – 1000hrs 1000- 1200hrs 1000-1400hrs	Lecture for final year BDS & Residents Lecture R3 to R2 (PAL) Demo: Ceph/Wire work/Cast (BDS) Clinical Work
Thursday	0830 – 0900hrs 9000-1000hrs 1100 – 1500hrs	CbD Lecture for final year BDS & Residents Treatment Planning Session & Discussion + Research Synopsis presentation
Friday	0800 – 0900hrs 0900 – 1200hrs	Lecture R4 to R3 (PAL) Lecture R2 to R1 (PAL) Wirework/Clinical Work

Chapter 21

LIST OF LOGISTICS FOR RESIDENTS

1.	Geometry Box
2.	Marking Pencil
3.	Acetate paper one pack
4.	Art pad and Graph Pad
5.	Vernier Caliper Digital with sharp beaks
6.	Cephalometric template
7.	Digital Camera
8.	Photographic mirror, Photo cheek retractors, Lip Retractors
9.	Stainless Steel Straight Wires (20 each)
	Round 0.014, 0.016, 0.018
	Rectangular 0.016X0.022, 0.017X0.025
10.	Laboratory Wires (1 Spool each) (0.5, 0.6, 0.7, 0.9) mm
11.	Laptop, USB, external hard drive and colour printer
12.	File cover and clear folders
13.	Brass wire
14.	ABO Ruler

List of Instruments

	Instruments	Quantity		Instruments	Quantity
1.	Hand piece	03	21.	How's pliers	01
2.	Metal Ruler in mm	10	22.	Tucker	06
3.	ABO scale	01	23.	Utility Instrument	06
4.	Wax knife	02	24.	Straight end cutter	06
5.	Plaster knife	02	25.	Distal end cutter	06
6.	Wax carver	02	26.	Torqueing pliers	02
7.	Periodontal probe	01	27.	Tweed loop forming pliers	01
8.	Dental Cheek Retractor C-shape (3 sizes)	03 each	28.	Step pliers	01
9.	Adam's pliers	01	29.	Turret	01
10.	Bird beak pliers light	02	30.	Examination set (Mouth mirror, Tweezer, Small probe)	10 sets
11.	Bird beak pliers heavy	01	31.	Fox occlusal plane	01
12.	Three prong pliers light	01	32.	Bracket positioning gauge	01
13.	Three prong pliers heavy	01	33.	Bracket holder	06
14.	Mathieu's pliers	10			
15.	Separator holding pliers	01			
16.	Band pusher	03			
17.	Band remover	03			
18.	Band seater	03			
19.	Bracket removing pliers	01			
20.	Weingart's pliers	06			

Chapter 22

ANNEXURES

ANNEXURE-1

Month
Year, 20

Mini Clinical Evaluation Exercise (Mini-CEX)								
It is mandatory for the trainee to get at least "Meets Expectations (3)" in the critical (highlighted) segment to pass								
Trainee:		**Assessor:** **Position:**						
Level of training Module I ____ II____ III ____ IV____ V ____ VI____ VII____VIII____								
Total Time: 10-15 Minutes		**Time for feedback: Minimum 5 minutes**						
Focus of encounter	**History** ☐	**Exam** ☐	**Evaluation** ☐		**Consent** ☐			
Please grade the following areas on the given scale*								
Attitudes		**1**	**2**	**3**	**4**	**5**	**NA**	
1.	Explaining the procedure before hand							
2.	Taking consent from the patient							
3.	Privacy of the patient							
4.	Comfort of the patient							
5.	Confidentiality of patient							
6.	**Confirms proper cross infection techniques performed during the whole procedure**							
	Remarks							
Skills		**1**	**2**	**3**	**4**	**5**	**NA**	
1.	**Clinical judgement & decision making**							
2.	**Communication & listening skills**							
3.	**History taking skills**							
4.	**Physical examination skills**							
5.	Organization & time management							
	Remarks							
Feedback: Verbal feedback is the compulsory constituent of this assessment. Please use this space to record areas of strength and weaknesses and suggestions for improvement.								
Date;	Trainee's signature:	Assessor's signature:						
Trainee's comments on this Mini-CEX Assessor's comments on this Mini-CEX								

* 1= Below Expectation, 2 = Border line, 3 = Meets Expectations, 4 = Good, 5 = Excellent, NA = Not Assessed

ANNEXURE-2

Month
Year, 20

Case-Based Discussion (CbD)							
It is mandatory for the trainee to get at least "Meets Expectations (3)" in the critical (highlighted) segment to pass							
Trainee:		**Assessor:** **Position:**					
Level of training Module I ____ II_____ III ____ IV____ V ____ VI____ VII____VIII____							
Total Time: 10 Minutes		**Time for feedback: Minimum 5 minutes**					
Case	Pre-Treatment ☐	Interim ☐	Post-Treatment ☐				
Focus of encounter	Record keeping ☐	Diagnosis ☐	Treatment plan ☐				
Status	Presenter ☐	Participant ☐					
Please grade the following areas on the given scale*							
	Assessment of presenter	**1**	**2**	**3**	**4**	**5**	**NA**
1.	Record keeping						
2.	Correctness of findings						
3.	Diagnostic skills & underlying knowledge base						
4.	**Treatment Planning**						
5.	Clinical judgement & decision making						
6.	Presentation skills						
7.	***Relevant investigations* e.g., Hand & wrist, PA Ceph, Occlusal, Periapical, CBCT, protrusive picture, Predication tracing, CO-CR etc.**						
	Remarks						
1.	Correctness of findings						
	Assessment of participant	**1**	**2**	**3**	**4**	**5**	**NA**
2.	Diagnostic skills & underlying knowledge base						
3.	**Treatment Planning**						
	Remarks						
Feedback: Verbal feedback is the compulsory constituent of this assessment. Please use this space to record areas of strength and weaknesses and suggestions for improvement.							
Date:	Trainee's signature:	Assessor's signature:					
Trainee's comments on this CbD Assessor's comments on this CbD							

* 1 = Below Expectation, 2 = Border line, 3 = Meets Expectations, 4 = Good, 5 = Excellent, NA = Not Assessed

ANNEXURE-3

			Month **Year, 20**				
Observation Of Teaching (OOT) Lecture/ Demonstration							
It is mandatory for the trainee to get at least "Meets Expectations (3)" in the critical (highlighted) segment to pass							
Trainee:		**Assessor:** **Position:**					
Level of training Module I ____ II_____ III ____ IV____ V ____ VI____ VII____VIII____							
Total Time: 30 Minutes		**Time for feedback: Minimum 5 minutes**					
Brief Description of Session:							
Please grade the following areas on the given scale*							
Attitudes		**1**	**2**	**3**	**4**	**5**	**NA**
1.	Communication						
2.	**Interaction**						
3.	Remarks						
Skills		**1**	**2**	**3**	**4**	**5**	**NA**
1.	Introduction & activation of prior knowledge						
2.	**Content**						
3.	**Presentation skills**						
4.	Conclusion						
	Remarks						
Feedback: Verbal feedback is the compulsory constituent of this assessment. Please use this space to record areas of strength and weaknesses and suggestions for improvement.							
Date:	Trainee's signature:	Assessor's signature:					
Trainee's comments on this OOT Assessor's comments on this OOT							

* 1 = Below Expectation, 2 = Border line, 3 = Meets Expectations, 4 = Good, 5 = Excellent, NA = Not Assessed

ANNEXURE-4

						Month **Year, 20**
Presentation ☐ **JCM** ☐ **PAL** ☐						
Observation Of Teaching (OOT)						
It is mandatory for the trainee to get at least "Meets Expectations (3)" in the critical (highlighted) segment to pass						
Trainee:			**Assessor:** **Position:**			
Level of training Module I ____ II____ III ____ IV____ V ____ VI____ VII____VIII____						
Total Time: 30 Minutes			**Time for feedback: Minimum 5 minutes**			
Brief Description of Session:						
Please grade the following areas on the given scale*						
Attitudes	**1**	**2**	**3**	**4**	**5**	**NA**
1. Communication						
2. **Interaction**						
Remarks						
Skills	**1**	**2**	**3**	**4**	**5**	**NA**
1. Introduction & activation of prior knowledge						
2. **Content**						
3. **Presentation skills**						
4. Conclusion						
Remarks						
Feedback: Verbal feedback is the compulsory constituent of this assessment. Please use this space to record areas of strength and weaknesses and suggestions for improvement.						
Date:	Trainee's signature:		Assessor's signature:			
Trainee's comments on this OOT Assessor's comments on this OOT						

* 1 = Below Expectation, 2 = Border line, 3 = Meets Expectations, 4 = Good, 5 = Excellent, NA = Not Assessed

ANNEXURE-5

Month	
Year, 20	

Patient Progress Proforma (PPP)	
It is mandatory for the trainee to get at least "Meets Expectations (3)" in the critical (highlighted) segment to be considered pass	
Trainee:	**Assessor:** **Position:**
Level of training: I ____ II____ III ____ IV____ V ____ VI____ VII____VIII____	
Total Time: 5 Minutes	**Time for feedback: Minimum 5 minutes**
Please grade the following areas on the given scale*	

		1	2	3	4	5	NA
1.	Complete background knowledge about the case						
2.	Proper case presentation at the appointment & highlights the relevant findings						
3.	Instruments available						
4.	Previous record complete and available						
5.	**Carries out previous instructions properly**						
6.	Explains the next treatment step along with its rationale						
7.	Proper management of "No show"/ "Missed appointment"						
8.	Manages difficult clinical situations properly (repeated bracket breakages, poor compliance etc.)						
9.	Shows any important treatment mechanics carried to the assessor						
10.	Shows empathetic attitude towards patient						
11.	Writes down the instructions given at each visit and shows it to the assessor after each appointment						
12.	**Manages time properly (Procedure time & schedule) and gives next appointment**						
	Remarks						

Feedback: Verbal feedback is the compulsory constituent of this assessment. Please use this space to record areas of strength and weaknesses and suggestions for improvement.		
Date:	Trainee's signature:	Assessor's signature:
Trainee's comments on this DOPS Assessor's comments on this DOPS		

* 1 = Below Expectation, 2 = Border line, 3 = Meets Expectations, 4 = Good, 5 = Excellent, NA = Not Assessed

ANNEXURE-6.1

Module I
Jan/Feb, 20

DOPS for Taking Impression and Wax bite (1) **It is mandatory for the trainee to get at least "Meets Expectations (3)" in the critical (highlighted) segment to clear this DOPS**							
Trainee:	**Assessor:** **Position:**						
Total Time: 15 Minutes	**Time for feedback: Minimum 5 minutes**						
Please grade the following areas on the given scale*							
	Attitudes	**1**	**2**	**3**	**4**	**5**	**NA**
1.	Explains the procedure before hand						
2.	Takes consent from the patient						
3.	Ensures privacy of the patient						
4.	Ensures comfort of the patient						
5.	Ensures confidentiality of the patient						
6.	Displays good communication during whole procedure						
7.	**Displays safe clinical practice during the whole procedure**						
8.	Exhibits high standards of professionalism during the whole procedure						
9.	**Adopts proper cross infection techniques during the whole procedure**						
10.	Gives proper reassurance if the patient is uncomfortable with the procedure						
	Remarks						
	Skills	**1**	**2**	**3**	**4**	**5**	**NA**
1.	Ensures proper instruments and materials are available						
2.	Chooses the suitable tray size						
3.	Checks the tray is properly loaded & positioned correctly in mouth						
4.	**Checks that impression is properly extended till the sulcus depth, no air bubble & all teeth are included in impression**						
5.	Takes a proper wax bite						
6.	Organizes proper disinfection of impressions and wax bite						
7.	Manages time properly						
	Remarks						

Feedback: Verbal feedback is the compulsory constituent of this assessment. Please use this space to record areas of strength and weaknesses and suggestions for improvement.		
Date:	Trainee's signature:	Assessor's signature:
Trainee's comments on this DOPS Assessor's comments on this DOPS		

* 1 = Below Expectation, 2 = Border line, 3 = Meets Expectations, 4 = Good, 5 = Excellent, NA = Not Assessed

ANNEXURE-6.2

Module I
March/April, 20

DOPS for Taking Impression and Wax bite (2) It is mandatory for the trainee to get at least "Meets Expectations (3)" in the critical (highlighted) segment to clear this DOPS							
Trainee:		**Assessor:** **Position:**					
Total Time: 15 minutes		**Time for feedback: Minimum 5 minutes**					
Please grade the following areas on the given scale*							
	Attitudes	**1**	**2**	**3**	**4**	**5**	**NA**
1.	Explains the procedure before hand						
2.	Takes consent from the patient						
3.	Ensures privacy of the patient						
4.	Ensures comfort of the patient						
5.	Ensures confidentiality of the patient						
6.	Displays good communication during whole procedure						
7.	**Displays safe clinical practice during the procedure**						
8.	Exhibits high standards of professionalism during the whole procedure						
9.	**Adopts proper cross infection techniques during the whole procedure**						
10.	Gives proper reassurance if the patient is uncomfortable with the procedure						
	Remarks						
	Skills	**1**	**2**	**3**	**4**	**5**	**NA**
1.	Ensures proper instruments and materials are available						
2.	Chooses the suitable tray size						
3.	Checks that the tray is properly loaded & positioned correctly in the mouth						
4.	**Checks that impression is properly extended till the sulcus depth, there is no air bubble and all teeth are included in the impression**						
5.	Takes a proper wax bite						
6.	Organizes proper disinfection of impressions & wax bite						
7.	Manages time properly						
	Remarks						

Feedback: Verbal feedback is the compulsory constituent of this assessment. Please use this space to record areas of strength and weaknesses and suggestions for improvement.

Date:	Trainee's signature:	Assessor's signature:

Trainee's comments on this DOPS

Assessor's comments on this DOPS

* 1 = Below Expectation, 2 = Border line, 3 = Meets Expectations, 4 = Good, 5 = Excellent, NA = Not Assessed

ANNEXURE-6.3

Module I **May/June, 20**

DOPS for Clinical Photography **It is mandatory for the trainee to get at least "Meets Expectations (3)" in the critical (highlighted) segment to clear this DOPS**							
Trainee:	**Assessor**: **Position:**						
Total Time: 15 minutes	**Time for feedback: Minimum 5 minutes**						
Please grade the following areas on the given scale*							
	Attitudes	**1**	**2**	**3**	**4**	**5**	**NA**
1.	Explains the procedure before hand						
2.	Takes consent from the patient						
3.	Ensures privacy of the patient						
4.	Ensures comfort of the patient						
5.	Ensures confidentiality of the patient						
6.	Displays good communication during whole procedure						
7.	Displays safe clinical practice during the whole procedure						
8.	Exhibits high standards of professionalism during the procedure						
9.	Adopts proper cross infection techniques during the whole procedure						
	Remarks						
	Skills	**1**	**2**	**3**	**4**	**5**	**NA**
1.	Ensures proper instruments and materials are available						
2.	Confirms that the patient is appropriately positioned for the extra and intra oral views						
3.	Displays accurate use of camera and flash for taking the extra oral and intra oral views						
4.	Confirms extra & Intra oral views at the correct magnification and properly focused, no saliva visible & no fogging of the mirror for the occlusal photographs						
5.	Manages time properly						
6.	Ensures photographs are uploaded onto the server						
7.	**Ensures that good quality photographs are printed on A4 page as per specifications of the department**						
	Remarks						
Feedback: Verbal feedback is the compulsory constituent of this assessment. Please use this space to record areas of strength and weaknesses and suggestions for improvement.							
Date:	Trainee's signature:	Assessor's signature:					
Trainee's comments on this DOPS Assessor's comments on this DOPS							

* 1 = Below Expectation, 2 = Border line, 3 = Meets Expectations, 4 = Good, 5 = Excellent, NA = Not Assessed

ANNEXURE-6.4

Module II July/August, 20

DOPS for TMJ Examination It is mandatory for the trainee to get at least "Meets Expectations (3)" in the critical (highlighted) segment to clear this DOPS							
Trainee:		**Assessor:** **Position:**					
Total Time: 15 minutes		**Time for feedback: Minimum 5 minutes**					
Please grade the following areas on the given scale*							
Attitudes		**1**	**2**	**3**	**4**	**5**	**NA**
1.	Explains the procedure before hand						
2.	Takes consent from the patient						
3.	Ensures privacy of the patient						
4.	Ensures comfort of the patient						
5.	Ensures confidentiality of the patient						
6.	Displays good communication during the procedure						
7.	Displays safe clinical practice during the whole procedure						
8.	Exhibits high standards of professionalism during the whole procedure						
9.	Adopts proper cross infection techniques during the whole procedure						
	Remarks						
Skills		**1**	**2**	**3**	**4**	**5**	**NA**
1.	Ensures proper instruments and materials are available						
2.	Confirms that the patient is appropriately positioned						
3.	Takes complete history for TMJ (Basic Screening Questions)						
4.	On Inspection, records facial asymmetry and jaw movements						
5.	**Palpates muscles** • Masseter • Temporalis • Sternocleiodomastiod • Posterior cervical						
6.	**Palpates the of TMJ** • **With mouth closed** • **During opening and closing** • **With the mouth fully open and fingers behind the condyle**						

Annexure-6.4 (Continued)

	Skills	**1**	**2**	**3**	**4**	**5**	**NA**
7.	**Checks functional manipulation of muscles during contracting & stretching** • **Lateral pterygoid (Inferior & Superior)** • **Medial pterygoid**						
8.	**Measures maximum incisal distance and records any deflection & deviation**						
9.	**Measures the protrusive and lateral mandibular movements**						
10.	Records TMJ Sounds						
11.	Manages time properly						
	Remarks						
Feedback: Verbal feedback is the compulsory constituent of this assessment. Please use this space to record areas of strength and weaknesses and suggestions for improvement.							
Date:	Trainee's signature:	Assessor's signature:					
Trainee's comments on this DOPS Assessor's comments on this DOPS							

* 1 = Below Expectation, 2 = Border line, 3 = Meets Expectations, 4 = Good, 5 = Excellent, NA = Not Assessed

ANNEXURE-6.5

Module II
Sep/Oct, 20

DOPS for Fitting Molar Bands **It is mandatory for the trainee to get at least "Meets Expectations (3)" in the critical (highlighted) segment to clear this DOPS**							
Trainee:	**Assessor:** **Position:**						
Total Time: 20 minutes (for one side upper & lower)	**Time for feedback: Minimum 5 minutes**						
Please grade the following areas on the given scale*							
	Attitudes	**1**	**2**	**3**	**4**	**5**	**NA**
1.	Explains the procedure before hand						
2.	Takes consent from the patient						
3.	Ensures privacy of the patient						
4.	**Ensures comfort of the patient**						
5.	Ensures confidentiality of the patient						
6.	Displays good communication during whole procedure						
7.	**Displays safe clinical practice during the whole procedure**						
8.	Exhibits high standards of professionalism during the procedure						
9.	**Adopts proper cross infection techniques during procedure**						
	Remarks						
	Skills	**1**	**2**	**3**	**4**	**5**	**NA**
1.	Ensures proper instruments and materials are available						
2.	Ensures the patient is positioned properly						
3.	Uses study cast as reference to estimate size. Removes separators & tries bands on teeth						
4.	Adopts the bands on tooth anatomy						
5.	Ensures band size is correct, flush with marginal ridges & equidistance						
6.	Removes, dries the band & blocks the slot with wax						
7.	Isolates the tooth & asks the assistant to apply cement in the band						
8.	Cements the bands in proper position in all dimensions and cleans excess cement and allows to set						
9.	Manages time properly						
10.	Confirm clinical records completed, follow-up appointment given						
	Remarks						

Feedback: Verbal feedback is the compulsory constituent of this assessment. Please use this space to record areas of strength and weaknesses and suggestions for improvement.		
Date:	Trainee's signature:	Assessor's signature:
Trainee's comments on this DOPS Assessor's comments on this DOPS		

* 1 = Below Expectation, 2 = Border line, 3 = Meets Expectations, 4 = Good, 5 = Excellent, NA = Not Assessed

ANNEXURE-6.6

Module II	
Nov/Dec, 20	

DOPS for Radiography (Lateral Ceph/OPG/Periapical/ Bitewing) It is mandatory for the trainee to get at least "Meets Expectations (3)" in the critical (highlighted) segment to clear this DOPS							
Trainee:	**Assessor: Position:**						
Total Time: 5-10 minutes	**Time for feedback: Minimum 5 Minutes**						
Please grade the following areas on the given scale*							
	Attitudes	**1**	**2**	**3**	**4**	**5**	**NA**
1.	Explains the procedure before hand						
2.	Takes consent from the patient						
3.	Ensures privacy of the patient						
4.	Ensures comfort of the patient						
5.	Ensures confidentiality of the patient						
6.	Displays good communication during whole procedure						
7.	**Displays safe clinical practice during whole procedure**						
8.	Exhibits high standards of professionalism during the whole procedure						
9.	Adopts proper cross infection techniques during the whole procedure						
	Skills	**1**	**2**	**3**	**4**	**5**	**NA**
1.	Ensures proper instruments and materials are available						
2.	Loads the film in the cassette or film holder						
3.	Ensures proper protective equipment is present (lead apron for patient & operator)						
4.	Places the lead apron fully, clearing the back of the neck region; high in front, low in back						
5.	Gives instructions to remove facial jewellery in the beam path (nose rings or large earrings), eyeglasses and intraoral prostheses.						
6.	Positions the patient (e.g., ear rods, Nasion pointer, chin rest and bite block) properly						
7.	Ensures patients head is in the focal trough						
8.	Ensures milliamperage and kilovoltage on control panel are according to specification						
9.	Gives instructions/ensures that the patient is appropriately positioned (Natural Head Position)						
10.	Gives pre-exposure instructions: positioning of the tongue and lips and remaining still during the entire exposure cycle.						
11.	Uses film holder where required (periapical/bitewing) and places the film properly						
12.	Properly angulates the cone for bisecting angle technique according to the tooth						

Annexure-6.6 (Continued)

	Skills	1	2	3	4	5	NA
13.	Ensures proper patient, film and cone distance						
14.	Stands at proper distance during exposure						
15.	Informs the patient before exposure to avoid sudden movement during exposure						
16.	Properly handles the film/cassette & transfer it to dark room						
17.	Follows all steps of film development (developing, fixing and drying) in sequence and for the required time						
18.	**Ensures film is properly developed (checks for any artefacts), showing the required field of vision and repeats it if necessary**						
19.	Manages time properly						
20.	Ensures that radiograph is properly labeled						
	Remarks						

Feedback: Verbal feedback is the compulsory constituent of this assessment. Please use this space to record areas of strength and weaknesses and suggestions for improvement.

Date:	Trainee's signature:	Assessor's signature:

Trainee's comments on this DOPS
Assessor's comments on this DOPS

* 1 = Below Expectation, 2 = Border line, 3 = Meets Expectations, 4 = Good, 5 = Excellent, NA = Not Assessed

ANNEXURE-6.7

Module III **Jan/Feb, 20**

DOPS for Bracket Bonding **It is mandatory for the trainee to get at least "Meets Expectations (3)" in the critical (highlighted) segment to clear this DOPS**							
Trainee:		**Assessor:** **Position:**					
Total Time: 15 minutes		**Time for feedback: Minimum 5 minutes**					
Please grade the following areas on the given scale*							
Attitudes		**1**	**2**	**3**	**4**	**5**	**NA**
1.	Explains the procedure before hand						
2.	Takes consent from the patient						
3.	Ensures privacy of the patient						
4.	Ensures comfort of the patient						
5.	Ensures confidentiality of the patient						
6.	Displays good communication during whole procedure						
7.	**Displays safe clinical practice during the whole procedure**						
8.	Exhibits high standards of professionalism during procedure						
9.	**Adopts proper cross infection techniques**						
	Remarks						
Skills		**1**	**2**	**3**	**4**	**5**	**NA**
1.	Ensures proper instruments and materials are available						
2.	Ensures proper protective equipment is present						
3.	Confirms that the patient is appropriately positioned						
4.	Ensures materials used safely and handled properly						
5.	Ensures any unpleasant incident dealt with properly						
6.	**Displays correct handling, placement & positioning of brackets**						
7.	Inverts or swaps brackets if necessary						
8.	Displays proper removal of excess bonding material (flash)						
9.	Manages time properly						
10.	Confirms clinical records completed & follow-up appointment given						
	Remarks						

Feedback: Verbal feedback is the compulsory constituent of this assessment. Please use this space to record areas of strength and weaknesses and suggestions for improvement.		
Date:	Trainee's signature:	Assessor's signature:
Trainee's comments on this DOPS Assessor's comments on this DOPS		

* 1 = Below Expectation, 2 = Border line, 3 = Meets Expectations, 4 = Good, 5 = Excellent, NA = Not Assessed

ANNEXURE-6.8

Module III	
March/April, 20	

DOPS for Fitting a Removable Functional Appliance **It is mandatory for the trainee to get at least "Meets Expectations (3)" in the critical (highlighted) segment to clear this DOPS**							
Trainee:		**Assessor:** **Position:**					
Total Time: 10 minutes		**Time for feedback: Minimum 5 minutes**					
Please grade the following areas on the given scale*							
Attitudes		**1**	**2**	**3**	**4**	**5**	**NA**
1.	Explains the procedure before hand						
2.	Takes consent from the patient						
3.	Ensures privacy of the patient						
4.	Ensures comfort of the patient						
5.	Ensures confidentiality of the patient						
6.	Displays good communication during whole procedure						
7.	**Displays safe clinical practice during the whole procedure**						
8.	Exhibits high standards of professionalism during the whole procedure						
9.	**Adopts proper cross infection techniques during the whole procedure**						
	Remarks						
Skills		**1**	**2**	**3**	**4**	**5**	**NA**
1.	Ensures proper instruments and materials are available						
2.	Ensures that the patient is positioned appropriately						
3.	Tries the functional appliance in mouth & confirms its retention						
4.	**Checks the mandibular posture and midline after insertion. Adjusts if necessary**						
5.	**Shows the insertion and removal technique to the patient by the help of face mirror**						
6.	Shows the patient how to open up the expansion screw if present & asks the patient to exercise						
7.	Ensures patient is expert at insertion & removal of appliance						
8.	**Describes care of appliance, e.g. hours of wear, handling during contact sports or swimming, cleaning of appliance, managing speech interference etc.**						
9.	Asks the patient to report back in cases of difficulties with wear, damage or loss of appliance						

Annexure-6.8 (Continued)

Skills		1	2	3	4	5	NA
10.	Ensures statement of compliance is signed and copy given to patient						
11.	Ensures base line clinical findings (overjet, overbite & molar relationship) are recorded at the insertion day						
12.	Manages time properly						
13.	Confirms clinical records are completed and follow-up appointment given						
	Remarks						
Feedback: Verbal feedback is the compulsory constituent of this assessment. Please use this space to record areas of strength and weaknesses and suggestions for improvement.							
Date:	Trainee's signature:	Assessor's signature:					
Trainee's comments on this DOPS Assessor's comments on this DOPS							

* 1 = Below Expectation, 2 = Border line, 3 = Meets Expectations, 4 = Good, 5 = Excellent, NA = Not Assessed

ANNEXURE-6.9

Module III	
May/June, 20	

DOPS for Orthodontic Mini-Implant Insertion **It is mandatory for the trainee to get at least "Meets Expectations (3)" in the critical (highlighted) segment to clear this DOPS**							
Trainee:	**Assessor:** **Position:**						
Total Time: 15 minutes	**Time for feedback: Minimum 5 minutes**						
Please grade the following areas on the given scale*							
	Attitudes	**1**	**2**	**3**	**4**	**5**	**NA**
1.	Explains the procedure before hand						
2.	Takes consent from the patient						
3.	Ensures privacy of the patient						
4.	Ensures comfort of the patient						
5.	Ensures confidentiality of the patient						
6.	Displays good communication during whole procedure						
7.	**Displays safe clinical practice during the whole procedure**						
8.	Exhibits high standards of professionalism during the whole procedure						
9.	**Adopts proper cross infection techniques during the whole procedure**						
	Remarks						
	Skills	**1**	**2**	**3**	**4**	**5**	**NA**
1.	Ensures proper instruments, preop radiograph and mini-Implants of proper size are available						
2.	Gives few drops of LA & checks its efficacy						
3.	Incises mucosa where necessary. Perforates the cortical plate with a probe/drill, where necessary						
4.	Securely & properly attaches implant driver onto mini-implant						
5.	Ensures proper retraction at the insertion site						
6.	Correctly angulates implant driver at insertion site & starts slow controlled mini-implant insertion						
7.	Confirms there is no root contact by percussing adjacent teeth						
8.	**Confirms proper mini-implant insertion depth radiographically & confirms head projection clinically**						
9.	Loads mini-implant with the accurate force level						

Annexure-6.9 (Continued)

Skills		1	2	3	4	5	NA
10.	Manages time properly						
11.	Confirms clinical records are completed and follow-up appointment given						
	Remarks						
Feedback: Verbal feedback is the compulsory constituent of this assessment. Please use this space to record areas of strength and weaknesses and suggestions for improvement.							
Date:	Trainee's signature:	Assessor's signature:					
Trainee's comments on this DOPS Assessor's comments on this DOPS							

* 1 = Below Expectation, 2 = Border line, 3 = Meets Expectations, 4 = Good, 5 = Excellent, NA = Not Assessed

ANNEXURE-6.10

Module IV	**July/Aug, 20**

DOPS for Selection and placement of Arch wire It is mandatory for the trainee to get at least "Meets Expectations (3)" in the critical (highlighted) segment to clear this DOPS							
Trainee:		**Assessor: Position:**					
Total Time: 10 minutes		**Time for feedback: Minimum 5 minutes**					
Please grade the following areas on the given scale*							
Attitudes		**1**	**2**	**3**	**4**	**5**	**NA**
1.	Explains the procedure before hand						
2.	Takes consent from the patient						
3.	Ensures privacy of the patient						
4.	Ensures comfort of the patient						
5.	Ensures confidentiality of the patient						
6.	Displays good communication during whole procedure						
7.	**Displays safe clinical practice during the whole procedure**						
8.	Exhibits high standards of professionalism during the whole procedure						
9.	**Adopts proper cross infection techniques during the whole procedure**						
	Remarks						
Skills		**1**	**2**	**3**	**4**	**5**	**NA**
1.	Ensures proper instruments and materials are available						
2.	Ensures proper protective equipment is present						
3.	Confirms that the patient is appropriately positioned						
4.	Ensures materials used safely and handled properly						
5.	Ensures any unpleasant incident dealt with properly						
6.	Removes existing arch wire, ligatures and any auxiliaries using appropriate instruments						
7.	Disposes off contaminated ligatures, auxiliaries and existing arch wire safely; observing health, safety and infection control measures						
8.	**Evaluates current clinical situation and determines tooth movements required for next stage of treatment**						
9.	**Selects arch wire material and dimensions appropriate for the required tooth movements. Explains this choice to assessor**						

Annexure-6.10 (Continued)

Skills		1	2	3	4	5	NA
10.	Uses study models as reference to customize arch wire to patient's arch dimensions (where appropriate), estimates length of arch wire required and shortens ends using appropriate instruments						
11.	Places arch wire in patient's mouth, ligates using appropriate ligature technique, and includes any necessary auxiliaries						
12.	Cuts distal ends of arch wire to final length for patient comfort using appropriate instruments, disposing off sharps safely and asks patient to check for sharp/rough ends						
13.	Demonstrates new wire to patient and explains about discomfort						
14.	Manages time properly						
15.	Confirms clinical records are completed and follow-up appointment given						
	Remarks						
Feedback: Verbal feedback is the compulsory constituent of this assessment. Please use this space to record areas of strength and weaknesses and suggestions for improvement.							
Date:	Trainee's signature:	Assessor's signature:					
Trainee's comments on this DOPS Assessor's comments on this DOPS							

* 1 = Below Expectation, 2 = Border line, 3 = Meets Expectations, 4 = Good, 5 = Excellent, NA = Not Assessed

ANNEXURE-6.11

Module IV Sep/Oct, 20

DOPS for Piggyback wire It is mandatory for the trainee to get at least "Meets Expectations (3)" in the critical (highlighted) segment to clear this DOPS							
Trainee:	**Assessor:** **Position:**						
Total Time: 15 minutes	**Time for feedback: Minimum 5 minutes**						
Please grade the following areas on the given scale*							
	Attitudes	**1**	**2**	**3**	**4**	**5**	**NA**
1.	Explains the procedure before hand						
2.	Takes consent from the patient						
3.	Ensures privacy of the patient						
4.	Ensures comfort of the patient						
5.	Ensures confidentiality of the patient						
6.	Displays good communication during whole procedure						
7.	**Displays safe clinical practice during the whole procedure**						
8.	Exhibits high standards of professionalism						
9.	**Adopts proper cross infection techniques during the whole procedure**						
	Remarks						
	Skills	**1**	**2**	**3**	**4**	**5**	**NA**
1.	Ensures proper instruments & materials are available						
2.	Ensures proper protective equipment is present						
3.	Confirms that the patient is appropriately positioned						
4.	Ensures materials used safely and handled properly						
5.	Ensures any unpleasant incident dealt with properly						
6.	Removes existing arch wire, ligatures and any auxiliaries using appropriate instruments						
7.	Disposes off contaminated ligatures, auxiliaries and existing arch wire safely; observing health and safety and infection control measures						
8.	**Ensures adequate anchorage preparation has been done**						
9.	Evaluates current clinical situation and determines tooth movements required for next stage of treatment						
10.	**Ensures there is enough arch length (space) to permit de-rotation and alignment of the tooth (to be piggy backed)**						
11.	Ensures the bracket on the tooth to be aligned is as much in its final position as possible						

Annexure-6.11 (Continued)

	Skills	1	2	3	4	5	NA
12.	**Ensures there is adequate maintenance of the space created in the arch**						
13.	Selects arch wire material and dimensions appropriate for the required tooth movements. Explains this choice to assessor						
14.	Uses study models as reference to customize arch wire to patient's arch dimensions (where appropriate), estimates length of arch wire required and shortens ends using appropriate instruments						
15.	Cuts the piggy back wire according to size required						
16.	Places piggyback in the auxiliary slot and main arch wire in main slot in molar tube, ligates using appropriate ligature technique, and includes any necessary auxiliaries						
17.	Uses the wire tucker if tooth is severely malaligned						
18.	Cuts distal ends of archwires to final length for patient comfort using appropriate instruments, disposing off sharps safely, asks patient to check for sharp/rough ends						
19.	Demonstrates new wires to patient and explains about discomfort						
20.	Manages time properly						
21.	Confirms clinical records are completed and follow-up appointment given						
	Remarks						

Feedback: Verbal feedback is the compulsory constituent of this assessment. Please use this space to record areas of strength and weaknesses and suggestions for improvement.		
Date:	Trainee's signature:	Assessor's signature:
Trainee's comments on this DOPS Assessor's comments on this DOPS		

* 1 = Below Expectation, 2 = Border line, 3 = Meets Expectations, 4 = Good, 5 = Excellent, NA = Not Assessed

ANNEXURE-6.12

Module IV **Nov/Dec, 20**

DOPS for Insertion of Arch wire for Segmental Canine Retraction **It is mandatory for the trainee to get at least "Meets Expectations (3)"** **in the critical (highlighted) segment to clear this DOPS**							
Trainee:	**Assessor:** **Position:**						
Total Time: 10 minutes	**Time for feedback: Minimum 5 minutes**						
Please grade the following areas on the given scale*							
	Attitudes	**1**	**2**	**3**	**4**	**5**	**NA**
1.	Explains the procedure before hand						
2.	Takes consent from the patient						
3.	Ensures privacy of the patient						
4.	Ensures comfort of the patient						
5.	Ensures confidentiality of the patient						
6.	Displays good communication during whole procedure						
7.	**Displays safe clinical practice during the whole procedure**						
8.	Exhibits high standards of professionalism during the whole procedure						
9.	**Adopts proper cross infection techniques during the whole procedure**						
	Remarks						
	Skills	**1**	**2**	**3**	**4**	**5**	**NA**
1.	Ensures proper instruments and materials are available						
2.	Ensures proper protective equipment is present						
3.	Confirms that the patient is appropriately positioned						
4.	Ensures materials used safely and handled properly						
5.	Ensures any unpleasant incident dealt with properly						
6.	**Inserts the canine retraction arch wire to check length of the loop**						
7.	Makes sure it doesn't irritate the sulcus						
8.	Checks that mesial end is turned at right angle/checks that sleeve is inserted						
9.	Ensures that ligatures are placed on premolars and canine is steel tied						
10.	Ensures that loop is properly activated and cinched back/ Inserts and activates the power O						
11.	Manages time properly						

Annexure-6.12 (Continued)

Skills		1	2	3	4	5	NA
12.	Confirms clinical records are completed and follow-up appointment given						
	Remarks						
Feedback: Verbal feedback is the compulsory constituent of this assessment. Please use this space to record areas of strength and weaknesses and suggestions for improvement.							
Date:	Trainee's signature:	Assessor's signature:					
Trainee's comments on this DOPS Assessor's comments on this DOPS							

* 1 = Below Expectation, 2 = Border line, 3 = Meets Expectations, 4 = Good, 5 = Excellent, NA = Not Assessed

ANNEXURE-6.13

Module V	
Jan/Feb, 20	

DOPS for Anterior Retraction with bilateral Helices, Class I/II/III Retraction It is mandatory for the trainee to get at least "Meets Expectations (3)" in the critical (highlighted) segment to clear this DOPS							
Trainee:		**Assessor:** **Position:**					
Total Time: 15 minutes		**Time for feedback: Minimum 5 minutes**					
Please grade the following areas on the given scale*							
Attitudes		**1**	**2**	**3**	**4**	**5**	**NA**
1.	Explains the procedure before hand						
2.	Takes consent from the patient						
3.	Ensures privacy of the patient						
4.	Ensures comfort of the patient						
5.	Ensures confidentiality of the patient						
6.	Displays good communication during whole procedure						
7.	**Displays safe clinical practice during the whole procedure**						
8.	Exhibits high standards of professionalism						
9.	**Adopts proper cross infection techniques during the whole procedure**						
	Remarks						
Skills		**1**	**2**	**3**	**4**	**5**	**NA**
1.	Ensures proper instruments and materials are available						
2.	Ensures proper protective equipment is present						
3.	Confirms that the patient is appropriately positioned						
4.	Ensures materials used safely and handled properly						
5.	Ensures any unpleasant incidents dealt with properly						
6.	Examines the patient if he/she requires anterior intrusion with retraction & informs this to assessor						
7.	**Chooses proper wire and explains to the assessor about the selection of arch wire. Marks distal to the lateral incisors**						
8.	**Makes helices with a proper pliers at the marked position**						
9.	Checks and modifies the arch form on the template/model according to the patients arch form						
10.	Incorporates anchor bends if anterior intrusion is also required						

Annexure-6.13 (Continued)

Skills		1	2	3	4	5	NA
11.	Cuts the extra length of the wire according to the patient arch & inserts the arch wire						
12.	**Ensures the proper positioning of the helices after insertion**						
13.	Inserts and activates the power O/Tieback properly for Class I traction Measures the elastics for Class II or III traction, selects the appropriate size & explains to assessor Directs/instructs/demonstrates to the patient & counsels for compliance						
14.	Tucks in the sharp end of ligature wire properly						
15.	Ensures the ligatures are placed and extra wire distal to molar tube is cut/cinched back						
16.	Manages time properly						
17.	Confirms clinical records are completed and follow-up appointment given						
	Remarks						

Feedback: Verbal feedback is the compulsory constituent of this assessment. Please use this space to record areas of strength and weaknesses and suggestions for improvement.		
Date:	Trainee's signature:	Assessor's signature:
Trainee's comments on this DOPS Assessor's comments on this DOPS		

* 1 = Below Expectation, 2 = Border line, 3 = Meets Expectations, 4 = Good, 5 = Excellent, NA = Not Assessed

ANNEXURE-6.14

Module V
March/April, 20

DOPS for Circumferential Supracrestal Fiberotomy (CSF) /Frenectomy/Gingivectomy or Gingivoplasty **It is mandatory for the trainee to get at least "Meets Expectations (3)" in the critical (highlighted) segment to clear this DOPS**							
Trainee:	**Assessor:** **Position:**						
Total Time:	**Time for feedback: Minimum 5 minutes**						
Please grade the following areas on the given scale*							
	Attitudes	**1**	**2**	**3**	**4**	**5**	**NA**
1.	Explains the procedure before hand						
2.	Takes consent from the patient						
3.	Ensures privacy of the patient						
4.	Ensures comfort of the patient						
5.	Ensures confidentiality of the patient						
6.	Displays good communication during whole procedure						
7.	**Displays safe clinical practice during the whole procedure**						
8.	Exhibits high standards of professionalism during the whole procedure						
9.	**Adopts proper cross infection techniques during the whole procedure**						
	Skills	**1**	**2**	**3**	**4**	**5**	**NA**
1.	Ensures proper instruments & materials available, like Local Anesthesia, blade #12,15, currettes, cotton rolls, pocket marker, artery forcep etc.						
2.	Ensures proper protective equipment is present						
3.	Confirms that the patient is appropriately positioned						
4.	Ensures materials used safely and handled properly						
5.	Ensures any unpleasant incident dealt with properly						
6.	Gives Local Anesthesia & checks its efficacy						
7.	Removes the Archwire and /marks the gingiva to be excised in case of gingivectomy by pocket marker						
8.	**Procedure:For *CSF* incises the supracrestal fibers properly from the labial side from interdental area & lingual side using blade #12/ performs *frenectomy* with blade # 15 a narrow elliptical incision around the frenal area down to the periosteum/for *gingivectomy* incision** should be beveled at approx. 45° to tooth surface to follow the scalloped outline of the gingiva						
9.	Maintains proper hemostatic control						

Annexure-6.14 (Continued)

Skills		1	2	3	4	5	NA
10.	Suturing/Pack: In ***frenectomy*** first interrupted suture should be at the maximal depth of the vestibule & should include both edges of mucosa & underlying periosteum at the height of the vestibule (reduces hematoma formation & adaptation of tissue to the maximal height of the vestibule)/In ***gingivectomy*** gives the periodontal pack if necessary						
11.	Gives proper instructions after the procedure and medicates if required						
12.	Manages time properly						
	Remarks						

Feedback: Verbal feedback is the compulsory constituent of this assessment. Please use this space to record areas of strength and weaknesses and suggestions for improvement.		
Date:	Trainee's signature:	Assessor's signature:
Trainee's comments on this DOPS Assessor's comments on this DOPS		

* 1 = Below Expectation, 2 = Border line, 3 = Meets Expectations, 4 = Good, 5 = Excellent, NA = Not Assessed

ANNEXURE-6.15

Module V
May/June, 20

DOPS for Face Bow Recording **It is mandatory for the trainee to get at least "Meets Expectations (3)" in the critical (highlighted) segment to clear this DOPS**							
Trainee:		**Assessor:** **Position:**					
Total Time: 15 minutes		**Time for feedback: Minimum 5 minutes**					
Please grade the following areas on the given scale*							
Attitudes		**1**	**2**	**3**	**4**	**5**	**NA**
1.	Explains the procedure before hand						
2.	Takes consent from the patient						
3.	Ensures privacy of the patient						
4.	Ensures comfort of the patient						
5.	Ensures confidentiality of the patient						
6.	Displays good communication during whole procedure						
7.	**Displays safe clinical practice during the whole procedure**						
8.	Exhibits high standards of professionalism during the whole procedure						
9.	**Adopts proper cross infection techniques during the whole procedure**						
	Remarks						
Skill		**1**	**2**	**3**	**4**	**5**	**NA**
1.	Ensures proper instruments and materials are available						
2.	Ensures proper protective equipment is present						
3.	Confirms that the patient is appropriately positioned						
4.	Ensures materials used safely and handled properly						
5.	Ensures any unpleasant incidents dealt with properly						
6.	Marks reference point on ala tragus line 13 mm ahead of tragus of ear on both sides						
7.	Ensures that bite fork is loaded with impression material and positioned correctly on maxillary occlusal plane						
8.	Ensures that ear rods correctly positioned (may need to be modified for facial asymmetry patients) on the reference marks and centered						
9.	**Ensures that the readings on both sides of ear rods are same and screws tightened**						

Annexure-6.15 (Continued)

Skills		1	2	3	4	5	NA
10.	**Reference point: Ensures that orbital reference pointer correctly positioned at inferior orbital foramen (Palpates the infraorbital border of the orbit and identifies the infraorbital foramen)**						
11.	**Ensures that bite forks correctly positioned on the transfer jig**						
12.	**Ensures transfer jig correctly positioned, parallel to interpupillary line and centered**						
13.	**Ensures that thumb screws tightened after slight forward pressure on facebow**						
14.	**Asks the patient/ assistant to support the facebow while s/he confirms all components are fixed in place**						
15.	**Before removal from the mouth, ensures transfer jig and bite fork screws fully tightened**						
16.	**Ensures to mount the face bow on the articulator in proper position**						
17.	Manages time properly						
18.	Confirms clinical records are completed and follow-up appointment given						
	Remarks						

Feedback: Verbal feedback is the compulsory constituent of this assessment. Please use this space to record areas of strength and weaknesses and suggestions for improvement.

Date:	Trainee's signature:	Assessor's signature:

Trainee's comments on this DOPS

Assessor's comments on this DOPS

* 1 = Below Expectation, 2 = Border line, 3 = Meets Expectations, 4 = Good, 5 = Excellent, NA = Not Assessed

ANNEXURE-6.16

Module VI
Jan/Feb, 20

DOPS for Anterior Retraction with bilateral Retraction Loops It is mandatory for the trainee to get at least "Meets Expectations (3)" in the critical (highlighted) segment to clear this DOPS							
Trainee:		**Assessor:** **Position:**					
Total Time: 10 minutes		**Time for feedback: Minimum 5 minutes**					
Please grade the following areas on the given scale*							
Attitudes		**1**	**2**	**3**	**4**	**5**	**NA**
1.	Explains the procedure before hand						
2.	Takes consent from the patient						
3.	Ensures privacy of the patient						
4.	Ensures comfort of the patient						
5.	Ensures confidentiality of the patient						
6.	Displays good communication during whole procedure						
7.	**Displays safe clinical practice during the whole procedure**						
8.	Exhibits high standards of professionalism						
9.	**Adopts proper cross infection techniques during the whole procedure**						
	Remarks						
Skills		**1**	**2**	**3**	**4**	**5**	**NA**
1.	Ensures proper instruments and materials are available						
2.	Ensures proper protective equipment is present						
3.	Confirms that the patient is appropriately positioned						
4.	Ensures materials used safely and handled properly						
5.	Ensures any unpleasant incident dealt with properly						
6.	Examines the patient if he/she requires anterior retraction with/without intrusion and informs this to the assessor						
7.	Chooses proper wire and explains to the assessor about the selection of arch wire. Marks distal to the lateral incisors						
8.	Makes retraction loops of appropriate height with proper pliers at the marked position with/without a step						
9.	**Checks and adapts the arch form on the template/model according to the patients arch form**						

Annexure-6.16 (Continued)

Skills		1	2	3	4	5	NA
11.	**Inserts the arch wire & confirms the height & position of loops, makes sure they do not irritate the sulcus**						
12.	Activates the loops and cinches back distal to the molar tube						
13.	Manages time properly						
14.	Confirms clinical records are completed and follow-up appointment given						
	Remarks						
Feedback: Verbal feedback is the compulsory constituent of this assessment. Please use this space to record areas of strength and weaknesses and suggestions for improvement.							
Date:	Trainee's signature:	Assessor's signature:					
Trainee's comments on this DOPS Assessor's comments on this DOPS							

* 1 = Below Expectation, 2 = Border line, 3 = Meets Expectations, 4 = Good, 5 = Excellent, NA = Not Assessed

ANNEXURE-6.17

				Module VI **March/April, 20**			
DOPS for Crimpable Hook/ Ball stops **It is mandatory for the trainee to get at least "Meets Expectations (3)" in the critical (highlighted) segment to be considered pass in this DOPS**							
Trainee:		**Assessor:** **Position:**					
Total Time: 10 minutes		**Time for feedback: Minimum 5 minutes**					
Please grade the following areas on the given scale:							
Attitudes		**1**	**2**	**3**	**4**	**5**	**NA**
1.	Explains the procedure before hand						
2.	Takes consent from the patient						
3.	Ensures privacy of the patient						
4.	Ensures comfort of the patient						
5.	Ensures confidentiality of the patient						
6.	Displays good communication during whole procedure						
7.	**Displays safe clinical practice during the whole procedure**						
8.	Exhibits high standards of professionalism during the whole procedure						
9.	Adopts proper cross infection techniques during the whole procedure						
	Remarks						
Skills		**1**	**2**	**3**	**4**	**5**	**NA**
1.	Ensures proper instruments and materials are available						
2.	Ensures proper protective equipment is present						
3.	Confirms that the patient is appropriately positioned						
4.	Ensures materials used safely and handled properly						
5.	Ensures any unpleasant incident dealt with properly						
6.	Selects the proper wire & inserts it						
7.	**Places the hook/shim/ball stop in proper position and crimps it with proper pliers**						
8.	**Checks that it is immobile**						
9.	Manages time properly						

Annexure-6.17 (Continued)

Skills		1	2	3	4	5	NA
10.	Confirms clinical records are completed and follow-up appointment given						
	Remarks						
Feedback: Verbal feedback is the compulsory constituent of this assessment. Please use this space to record areas of strength and weaknesses and suggestions for improvement.							
Date:	Trainee's signature:	Assessor's signature:					
Trainee's comments on this DOPS Assessor's comments on this DOPS							

* 1 = Below Expectation, 2 = Border line, 3 = Meets Expectations, 4 = Good, 5 = Excellent, NA = Not Assessed

ANNEXURE-6.18

Module VI **May/June, 20**	

DOPS for insertion of Distal Jet/ Jones Jig **It is mandatory for the trainee to get at least "Meets Expectations (3)" in the critical (highlighted) segment to clear this DOPS**	
Trainee	**Assessor:** **Position:**
Total Time: 15 minutes	**Time for feedback: Minimum 5 minutes**
Please grade the following areas on the given scale:	

	Attitudes	**1**	**2**	**3**	**4**	**5**	**NA**
1.	Explains the procedure before hand						
2.	Takes consent from the patient						
3.	Ensures privacy of the patient						
4.	Ensures comfort of the patient						
5.	Ensures confidentiality of the patient						
6.	Displays good communication during whole procedure						
7.	**Displays safe clinical practice during the whole procedure**						
8.	Exhibits high standards of professionalism						
9.	**Adopts proper cross infection techniques during the whole procedure**						
	Remarks						
	Skills	**1**	**2**	**3**	**4**	**5**	**NA**
1.	Ensures proper instruments and materials are available						
2.	Ensures proper protective equipment is present						
3.	Confirms that the patient is appropriately positioned						
4.	Ensures materials used safely & handled properly						
5.	Ensures any unpleasant incident dealt with properly						
6.	Makes sure acrylic button of distal jet is smooth						
7.	**Makes sure anchorage is reinforced by proper coverage of palate with acrylic button in distal jet/ Figure 8 from second premolar on one side to other in Jones jig. Inserts heavy arch wire**						

Annexure-6.18 (Continued)

Skills		1	2	3	4	5	NA
8.	**Ensures molar bands are cemented prior to insertion of appliance in Jones Jig, excess material removed & bands properly flushed/inserts appliance with molar & premolar bands in distal jet**						
9.	**Makes sure that proper size of spring is inserted**						
10.	**Tightens the screws in distal jet/ligate with ligature wire to molars and premolars in Jones Jig in order to activate**						
11.	Makes sure no part is impinging or irritating soft tissues/tucks in the sharp edges of ligature wire in jones jig						
12.	Manages time properly						
13.	Confirms clinical records are completed and follow-up appointment given						
	Remarks						

Feedback: Verbal feedback is the compulsory constituent of this assessment. Please use this space to record areas of strength and weaknesses and suggestions for improvement.		
Date:	Trainee's signature:	Assessor's signature:
Trainee's comments on this DOPS Assessor's comments on this DOPS		

* 1 = Below Expectation, 2 = Border line, 3 = Meets Expectations, 4 = Good, 5 = Excellent, NA = Not Assessed

ANNEXURE-6.19

Module VII
July/August, 20

DOPS for Finishing and Detailing **It is mandatory for the trainee to get at least "Meets Expectations (3)" in the critical (highlighted) segment to clear this DOPS**							
Trainee:		**Assessor:** **Position:**					
Total Time: 15 minutes		**Time for Feedback: Minimum 5 minutes**					
Please grade the following areas on the given scale:							
Attitudes		**1**	**2**	**3**	**4**	**5**	**NA**
1.	Explains the procedure before hand						
2.	Takes consent from the patient						
3.	Ensures privacy of the patient						
4.	Ensures comfort of the patient						
5.	Ensures confidentiality of the patient						
6.	Displays good communication during whole procedure						
7.	**Displays safe clinical practice during the whole procedure**						
8.	Exhibits high standards of professionalism during the whole procedure						
9.	**Performs proper cross infection techniques during the whole procedure**						
	Remarks						
Skills		**1**	**2**	**3**	**4**	**5**	**NA**
1.	**Makes sure all the spaces closed, canines in class I and heavy rectangular wire has been passed before the start of finishing. Explains the assessor finishing steps and sequence required on Models and OPG & identifies which of the following needs correction:**						
	Rotations						
	Tip						
	Torque						
	In-out,						
	Molar position						
	Molar Toe-in, Toe-out, Molar In, out						
	Midlines						
	Arch Coordination						
	Posterior settling						
	Smile consonance						
	Incisal show						

Annexure-6.19 (Continued)

Skills		1	2	3	4	5	NA
2.	Makes correct identification of any brackets that need repositioning						
3.	Makes correct identification of any wire bends that are needed						
4.	Selects appropriate arch wire/auxiliary & places it						
5.	Demonstrates appropriate placement of finishing bends in the archwire(s)						
6.	Gives appropriate instructions to the patients for the elastics etc.						
7.	Manages time properly						
8.	Confirms clinical records are completed and follow-up appointment given						
	Remarks						
Feedback: Verbal feedback is the compulsory constituent of this assessment. Please use this space to record areas of strength and weaknesses and suggestions for improvement.							
Date:	Trainee's signature:	Assessor's signature:					
Trainee's comments on this DOPS Assessor's comments on this DOPS							

* 1 = Below Expectation, 2 = Border line, 3 = Meets Expectations, 4 = Good, 5 = Excellent, NA = Not Assessed

ANNEXURE-6.20

Module VII	
Sep/Oct, 20	

DOPS for Indirect Bonding **It is mandatory for the trainee to get at least "Meets Expectations (3)" in the critical (highlighted) segment to clear this DOPS**							
Trainee:		**Assessor:** **Position:**					
Total Time: 20 minutes		**Time for Feedback: Minimum 5 minutes**					
Please grade the following areas on the given scale*							
	Attitudes	**1**	**2**	**3**	**4**	**5**	**NA**
1.	Explains the procedure before hand						
2.	Takes consent from the patient						
3.	Ensures privacy of the patient						
4.	Ensures comfort of the patient						
5.	Ensures confidentiality of the patient						
6.	Displays good communication during whole procedure						
7.	Displays safe clinical practice during the whole procedure						
8.	Exhibits high standards of professionalism during the whole procedure						
9.	**Performs proper cross infection techniques during the whole procedure**						
	Remarks						
	Skills	**1**	**2**	**3**	**4**	**5**	**NA**
1.	Polishes all the teeth						
2.	Shows the bonding trays to the patient and explains the procedure						
3.	Sections the trays if required						
4.	Isolates the teeth that are to be bonded						
5.	Dries the teeth thoroughly						
6.	Etches the teeth properly						
7.	Washes away the etching gel with suction and water jet, & makes sure saliva does not come into contact with the etched enamel						
8.	Makes sure to completely dry the teeth surface						
9.	Applies appropriate amount of Resin A on tooth surface and Resin B on bracket mesh in the bonding tray						
10.	Positions the tray on teeth and seats the tray with hinge motion, applies equal pressure on occlusal, labial and buccal surfaces						

Annexure-6.20 (Continued)

	Skills	**1**	**2**	**3**	**4**	**5**	**NA**
11.	Removes the tray carefully						
12.	**Makes sure that the brackets are properly positioned and bonded, there is no excess resin on the teeth. Flosses the interproximal contacts**						
	Remarks						

Feedback: Verbal feedback is the compulsory constituent of this assessment. Please use this space to record areas of strength and weaknesses and suggestions for improvement.		
Date:	Trainee's signature:	Assessor's signature:
Trainee's comments on this DOPS Assessor's comments on this DOPS		

* 1 = Below Expectation, 2 = Border line, 3 = Meets Expectations, 4 = Good, 5 = Excellent, NA = Not Assessed

ANNEXURE-6.21

Module VIII **July/Aug, 20**	

DOPS for Debonding and Retention **It is mandatory for the trainee to get at least "Meets Expectations (3)" in the critical (highlighted) segment to clear this DOPS**							
Trainee:		**Assessor:** **Position:**					
Total Time: 30 minutes		**Time for Feedback: Minimum 5 minutes**					
Please grade the following areas on the given scale*							
Attitudes		**1**	**2**	**3**	**4**	**5**	**NA**
1.	Explains the procedure before hand						
2.	Takes consent from the patient						
3.	Ensures privacy of the patient						
4.	Ensures comfort of the patient						
5.	Ensures confidentiality of the patient						
6.	Displays good communication during whole procedure						
7.	**Displays safe clinical practice during the whole procedure**						
8.	Exhibits high standards of professionalism						
9.	**Performs proper cross infection techniques during the whole procedure**						
	Remarks						
Skills		**1**	**2**	**3**	**4**	**5**	**NA**
1.	Ensures proper instruments and materials are available						
2.	Ensures proper protective equipment is present						
3.	Confirms that the patient is appropriately positioned						
4.	Ensures materials used safely and handled properly						
5.	Ensures any unpleasant incidents dealt with properly						
6.	**Debonds the brackets by squeezing the bracket wings mesiodistally & lifts the bracket off with peel force /grips the bracket and lifts them off with 45° angle with proper pliers**						
7.	**Removes the bands with band remover by applying pressure primarily by engaging the band remover from the palatal side for maxillary arch and from buccal side for mandibular arch**						
8.	Removes the residual adhesive from the tooth surface by using appropriate bur with water spray						
9.	Dries the surface to see if adhesive is still present						
10.	**Ensures that all the adhesive is removed from enamel and** remains careful not to damage enamel						
11.	**Polishes the surfaces of all the teeth**						

Annexure-6.21 (Continued)

Skills		1	2	3	4	5	NA
12.	Takes proper impression with alginate						
13.	Sends the patient for scaling						
	Fixed Retainer						
1.	Makes sure lingual surface is cleaned before starting the procedure						
2.	Contours the wire on the lingual side of all the anterior teeth						
3.	Ensures appropriate moisture control						
4.	**Ensures correct retainer wire handling and placement/positioning**						
5.	Ensures correct application of etching and bonding agent by first tacking and then bulk of adhesive placement						
6.	**Ensures appropriate application and curing of bonding material with curing light and appropriate protection for operator/patient/ assistant**						
7.	Ensures appropriate removal of any excess bonding material with appropriate bur and checks occlusion						
8.	Demonstrates new bonded retainer to the patient and explains about oral hygiene and future care						
9.	Manages time properly						
10.	Confirms clinical records are completed and follow-up appointment given						
	Removable Retainer						
1.	Checks the retainer fabrication on model						
2.	**Tries the removable retainer in patients mouth and checks for fit, extension and retention.**						
3.	Ask the patient to try the appliance so as to know if he/she has understood insertion and removal						
4.	Gives proper instructions regarding wear of appliance						
5.	Demonstrates the retainer to the patient and explains cleaning of retainer and future care						
6.	Confirms clinical records are completed and follow-up appointment given						
	Remarks						

Feedback: Verbal feedback is the compulsory constituent of this assessment. Please use this space to record areas of strength and weaknesses and suggestions for improvement.

Date:	Trainee's signature:	Assessor's signature:

Trainee's comments on this DOPS
Assessor's comments on this DOPS

* 1 = Below Expectation, 2 = Border line, 3 = Meets Expectations, 4 = Good, 5 = Excellent, NA = Not Assessed

ANNEXURE-6.22

Module VIII Sep/Oct, 20

DOPS for Disciplinary Procedures It is mandatory for the trainee to get at least "Meets Expectations (3)" in the critical (highlighted) segment to clear this DOPS	
Trainee:	**Assessor:** **Position:**
Total Time: 15- 30 minutes	**Time for Feedback: Minimum 5 minutes**
Please grade the following areas on the given scale*	

	Attitudes	**1**	**2**	**3**	**4**	**5**	**NA**
1.	Listens to the complaint carefully						
2.	Investigates/gathers all findings carefully						
3.	Ensures privacy						
4.	Listens to both sides						
5.	Asks for any witnesses, gathers new evidence						
6.	Gathers all findings carefully						
7.	Seeks help from colleagues/ seniors/ supervisor where necessary						
8.	Documents the incidence where necessary						
9.	Gives Clear reason of his/her decision						
10.	Ensures to be reasonable, ensures due action matches the misconduct						
11.	**Shows patience, reflects, considers and then decides**						
12.	Gives verbal warning /written notification						
13.	Displays good communication during whole procedure						
14.	Exhibits high standards of professionalism						
	Remarks						

Feedback: Verbal feedback is the compulsory constituent of this assessment. Please use this space to record areas of strength and weaknesses and suggestions for improvement.

Date:	Trainee's signature:	Assessor's signature:
Trainee's comments on this DOPS Assessor's comments on this DOPS		

* 1 = Below Expectation, 2 = Border line, 3 = Meets Expectations, 4 = Good, 5 = Excellent, NA = Not Assessed

Chapter 23

Log Book

Module I

This log book covers all the cephalometric analyses, growth prediction, cast analysis, space analysis, mixed dentition analysis, Bolton analysis and indices to be covered during the first six months of training

Attach Lateral Cephalometric tracing here and identify the landmarks:

Landmarks of Lateral Cephalogram [9-11]

Sr No.	Landmarks; Hard Tissue	Abbreviations
1	Anterior Nasal Spine	ANS/Ans
2	Anterior point of the occlusal plane	APOcc
3	Articulare	Ar/ar
4	Basion	Ba
5	Bolton	Bo
6	Condylion	Cd
7	Coronoid	Cor
8	Glabella	Gl/G
9	Gonion	Go/go
10	Gnathion	Gn/gn
11	Incisor inferioris	Ii
12	Incisor superioris	Is
13	Infradentale	Id
14	Mandibular central incisor	LI/L1
15	Mandibular first molar	L6
16	Maxillary central incisor	UI/U1
17	Maxillary first molar	U6
18	Menton	Me/M
19	Nasion	N/Na
20	Orbitale	Or
21	Posterior Nasal Spine	PNS/Pns
22	Pogonion	Pog/Pg
23	Point A- subspinale	A
24	Point B- supramentale	B

(This page is intentionally left blank)

Sr No.	Landmarks; Hard Tissue	Abbreviations
25	Porion	Po
26	Posterior point for the occlusal plane	PPOcc
27	Prosthion (supradentale)	Pr
28	Pterygomaxillary fissure	Ptm/PTM
29	Sella	S
30	Sphenoethimoidale	SE
31	Spheno-occipital synchondrosis	SO
	Landmarks; Soft Tissue	
32	Glabella	G'
33	Nasion	N'/Ns
34	Pronasale	Pn/Cm(COGS)
35	Subnasale	Sn
36	Superior labial sulcus	Sls
37	Labrale superioris	Ls'
38	Stomion superioris	Sts/Stm_s
39	Stomion	St/Stm
40	Stomion inferioris	Sti/Stm_i
41	Labrale inferioris	Li'
42	Inferior labial sulcus	Ils
43	Pogonion	Pog'/Pos
44	Menton	Me'/Ms

Attach Lateral Cephalometric tracing here and draw the planes:

Planes of Lateral Cephalogram [9-11]

Sr No.	Planes; Lateral Cephalogram	Abbreviations
1	Sella Nasion plane (SN)	S-N
2	Frankfort horizontal plane (FH)	Or-Po
3	Palatal plane (PP or Pal)	ANS-PNS
4	Occlusal plane (Occ or OP)	APOcc-PPOcc
5	Mandibular plane (MP)	Me-Go
6	Gonion Gnathion plane	Go-Gn
7	Huxley's plane	Na-Ba
8	Facial plane	Na-Pog
9	Ricketts Esthetic line (E-line or EL)	Pn-Pog'
10	Ramal plane	Ar-Go
11	A-Pogonion line	A-Pog
12	Margoli's line	N-SO
13	Stiener line (S-line)	Cm-Pog'
14	Holdaway line (H-line)	Ls-Pog'
15	Burstone line (B-line)	Sn-Pog'

Attach Lateral Cephalometric tracing here and do Eastman Correction:

Eastman Correction [12, 13]

Eastman correction can be applied if SNA is high/low and SN/MxP is normal (5°-11°). This corrects for aberrant position of Nasion, assuming Sella is correct.

Correction of ANB:

1. Measured SNA= ______________
2. Measured SNB= ______________
3. ANB = ______________

$$\textbf{Corrected ANB (X)} = \frac{\textbf{Measured SNA - Average SNA (82)}}{\textbf{2}}$$

Eastman corrected ANB = measured ANB ± X

If SNA is higher than the average value (82) subtract X from ANB
If SNA is lower than the average value (82) add X to ANB
If SNA is higher than the average value (82) subtract X from ANB
If SNA is lower than the average value (82) add X from ANB

SNA > than 82°:

Eastman corrected ANB = X – measured ANB (_____- _____)

Corrected ANB = ________________

SNA < than 82°:

Eastman corrected ANB = X + measured ANB (_____+ _____)

Corrected ANB = ________________

Attach Cephalometric tracing here and do Cephalometric Correction (SN-FH Correction):

Cephalometric Correction (SN-FH Correction [14])

Before Correction

SNA = ______________

SNB = ______________

ANB = ______________

Draw the corrected plane 7 degree above SN plane, and measure new readings;

After Correction

SNA = ______________

SNB = ______________

ANB = ______________

Attach Lateral Cephalometric tracing here and do Wits Appraisal:

Wits Appraisal [15-19]

Reference value

Males: - 1mm Females: 0 mm

Patient's measurements:

____

Interpretation:

____

____

____

Attach Lateral Cephalometric tracing here and do Composite Analysis:

Composite Analysis [15, 17]

Sagittal analysis

1.	SNA	82 ± 2°	
2.	SNB	80 ± 2°	
3.	ANB	0 ± 4°	
4.	Wits	-1mm ♂ 0mm ♀	
5.	Anterior Cranial Base Length	(X)	
6.	Mandibular Corpus Length	(X + 7)	
7.	Facial Angle	81 ± 4°	

Dental analysis

1.	UI – SN	102 ± 5°	
2.	UI – Palatal	108 ± 5°	
3.	IMPA	90 ± 5°	
4.	I.I. A	135 ± 5°	
5.	UI– NA Distance	4mm	
6.	UI– NA Angle	22°	
7.	LI – NB Distance	4mm	
8.	LI – NB Angle	25°	
9.	Holdaway Ratio LI - NB:Pog- NB	1 : 1	
10.	LI- APog Line	0 mm	

Vertical analysis

1.	SN-Mand Plane	32 ± 4°	
2.	SN-Palatal Plane	6 ± 4°	
3.	SN-Occ Plane	17 ± 4°	
4.	MMA	25 ± 4°	
5.	Upper Occ	11 ± 4°	
6.	Lower Occ	14 ± 4°	
7.	Y – Axis	66 ± 4°	
8.	Sum of Posterior Angles (Saddle + Articulare + Gonial)	120° + 147° +120° = 396 ± 4°	
9.	PFH: AFH	65% ± 4%	
10.	LAFH: TAFH	54% ± 2%	

Soft tissue analysis

1.	Upper Lip to E Line	-3 mm ± 2 mm	
2.	Lower Lip to E Line	-2 mm ± 2 mm	
3.	Upper Lip to S Line	0 mm ± 2 mm	
4.	Lower Lip to S Line	0 mm ± 2 mm	
5.	Nasolabial Angle	102 ± 8°	

(This page is intentionally left blank)

Cephalometric Diagnosis

Sagittal: ____

Vertical: ____

Dental: ____

Soft Tissue: ____

Attach Lateral Cephalometric tracing here and do Wylie Analysis:

Wylie Analysis [15, 16, 20, 21]

Sr No.	Measurement	Reference	Patient's Readings	Difference	
				Orthognathic	Prognathic
1.	Glenoid Fossa to Sella	M = 18 mm F = 17 mm			
2.	Sella to Ptm	M = 18mm F = 17mm			
3.	Maxillary Length (ANS-PNS)	52 mm			
4.	Ptm to Buccal groove of upper 6	M = 15mm F = 16 mm			
5.	Mandibular Length	M = 103 mm F = 101 mm			
	Total				

Unit of Dysplasia = Prognathic- Orthognathic = -------------------
Class ---------------------------- tendency

Interpretation:

___

___

___

Attach Lateral Cephalometric tracing here and do Ricketts Analysis:

Ricketts Analysis [15-17]

Sr No.	Measurement	Mean ± SD	Patient's Readings
1.	Facial Angle Axis (Na-Ba- to CC-Gn)	90° ± 3	
2.	Facial Angle (N-Pog to FHP)	89° ± 3	
3.	Mandibular Plane Angle (MP-FHP)	26.0 ± 4.5	
4.	Mandibular Bend Angle	26° ± 4	
5.	Point A to Facial Plane	2 ± 2	
6.	PP to Frankfurt Plane	1°± 3.5	
7.	The Oral Gnomon	45°	
8.	LI to A-Pog Line (mm)	1mm ± 2	
9.	LI to A-Pog Line (angle)	22° ± 4	
10.	UI to A-Pog Line(mm)	1mm	
11.	UI to A-Pog Line (angle)	22°	
12.	Interincisal angle	125°	
13.	Maxillary 6 to Pterygoid Vertical Root	15mm (Age +3mm)	
14.	Lower lip to E- line	1mm	

Interpretation:

____

____

____

Attach Lateral Cephalometric tracing here and do Down's Analysis:

Down's Analysis [15-17]

Sr No.	Readings	Reference	Patient's Readings
1.	Facial Angle (FHP-NPg)	87.8° ± 3.6°	
2.	Angle of Convexity (N-A-Pg)	0° ± 5.1°	
3.	A-B-Plane Angle (AB-NPg)	-4.8° ± 3.7°	
4.	Mandibular Plane Angle (MnGo-FHP)	21.9° ±3.2^0	
5.	Y- Axis	59.4° ± 3.8°	
6.	Cant of occlusal plane (occlusal - FHP)	9.3° ± 3.8°	
7.	UI-LI (IIA)	135.4° ± 5.8°	
8.	LI to occlusal plane	14.5°±3.5	
9.	LI to Mandibular plane	1.4° ±3.8° (-8.5 to +7)	
10.	UI- AP Line	2.7mm ± 1.8mm	

Interpretation:

____

____

____

Attach Lateral Cephalometric tracing here and do Steiner Analysis:

Steiner Analysis [15-17, 22, 23]

Sr No.	Measurement	Mean + SD	Patient's Readings
1.	SNA	82° ± 2°	
2.	SNB	80° ± 2°	
3.	ANB	0-4°	
4.	SND	76°	
5.	UI to NA(mm)	4mm	
6.	UI to NA (°)	22°	
7.	LI to NB (mm)	4mm	
8.	LI to NB (°)	25°	
9.	Pog to NB	3mm	
10.	Holdaway Ratio LI - NB: Pog- NB	1:1	
11.	IIA	130°	
12.	SN to Occ	14°	
13.	SN to Go-Gn	32°	
14.	SL	51mm	
15.	SE	22mm	

Interpretation:

____

____

____

Attach Lateral Cephalometric Tracing here and draw Margoli's Triangle:

Margoli's Triangle [16]

Sr No.	Measurement	Mean + SD	Patient's Readings
1.	Craniofacial Angle (XNM)	72.8° ± 2.36°	
2.	Faciomandibular Angle (NMX)	67.4° ± 2.77°	
3.	Craniomandibular Angle (NXM)	39.6° ± 3.26°	

Interpretation:

____

____

____

Attach Lateral Cephalometric tracing here and do Tweed Analysis:

Tweed Analysis [17, 24-26]

Sr No.	Measurement	Abbreviation	Range	Patient's Readings
1.	Sella-Nasion-Point A	SNA	80-84°	
2.	Sella-Nasion-Point B	SNB	78-82°	
3.	Point A-Nasion-Point B	ANB	1-5°	
4.	Point A & Point B to occlusal plane	AO-BO	0-4mm	
5.	Occlusal plane	OP-FH	8-12°	
6.	Z-Angle	Z-Angle	75-78°	
7.	Upper lip thickness	UL		
8.	Total chin thickness	TC		
9.	Upper Lip thickness/Total Chin thickness	UL:TC	1:1	
10.	Anterior Facial Height/Posterior Facial Height ratio	AFH: PFH	0.65-0.75	

Interpretation:

____

____

____

Attach Lateral Cephalometric tracing here and draw Tweed Triangle:

Tweed Triangle [15, 16, 24-26]

Sr No.	Measurement	Reference	Patient's Readings
1.	FMA	25°	
2.	IMPA	90°	
3.	FMIA	65°	

FMA 21-29° =FMIA should be 68°

FMA >30° = FMIA should be 65°

If FMA is 20° or less, then IMPA should not exceed 92°

Interpretation:

____

____

____

Attach Lateral Cephalometric tracing here and do Columbia Analysis:

Columbia Analysis [16]

Sr No.	Measurement	Mean + SD (Adults)	Patient's Readings
1.	SNA	82° ± 3.9°	
2.	SNB	80° ± 3.6°	
3.	ANB	0-4°	
4.	SN to Go-Gn	31° ± 5.2°	
5.	Y-Axis (N-S-Gn)	67°	
6.	Holdaway Angle	7-8°	
7.	LI-GoGn	91.9° ± 7.6°	
8.	UI-SN	104°	
9.	Angle UI/LI	130°	
10.	Palatal to Go-Gn plane	22°±5.6°	
11.	LI-APog	0mm (-1 to +3)	
12.	LI-NB	4mm	
13.	NB-Pog	4mm	
14.	Holdaway Ratio LI-NB: NB-Pog	1:1	
15.	Jarabak Ratio S-Go/N-Me	0.65	
16.	Ratio N-ANS/ANS-Me	0.80	
17.	Extension of GoGn	+,0,-	

Interpretation:

___

___

___

Attach Lateral Cephalometric tracing here and do Sassouni Analysis:

Sassouni Analysis [15, 16, 27-29]

Facial Type:

____

Interpretation:

____

____

____

Attach Lateral Cephalometric tracing here and do Modified Sassouni Analysis:

Modified Sassouni Analysis [16, 27]

Facial type:

Profile type:

Diagnosis:

1. Evaluation of planes:
2. Evaluation of profile:
3. Anterior posterior relation:
4. Evaluation of position of maxillary molars:
5. Evaluation of posterior balance:
6. Size of corpus:
7. Vertical balance:
8. Vertical position of incisors:
9. Axial inclination of incisors

Attach Lateral Cephalometric tracing here and do McNamara Analysis:

COMPSITE NORMS		
Midfacial Length (mm) (Co-Pt. A)	**Mandibular Length (Co-Gn)**	**Lower Anterior Facial Height (mm) (ANS-Me)**
80	97-100	57-58
81	99-102	57-58
82	101-104	58-59
83	103-105	58-59
84	104-107	59-60
85	105-108	60-62
86	107-110	60-62
87	109-112	61-63
88	111-114	61-63
89	112-115	62-64
90	113-116	63-64
91	115-118	63-64
92	117-120	64-65
93	119-122	65-66
94	121-124	66-67
95	122-125	67-79
96	124-127	67-69
97	126-129	68-70
98	128-131	68-70
99	129-132	69-71
100	130-133	70-74
101	132-135	71-75
102	134-137	72-76
103	136-139	73-77
104	137-140	74-78
105	138-141	75-79

McNamara Analysis [15, 17, 30]

Sr No.	Measurement	Mean ± SD		Patient's Readings
		Female	Male	
Maxilla To Cranial Base				
1.	Nasion perpendicular – point A	0.4 ± 2.3mm	1.1 ± 2.7mm	
2.	SNA angle	82.4°± 3.0°	83.9°± 3.2°	
Mandible To Cranial Base				
3.	Nasion perpendicular-Pog	- 1.8 ± 4.5mm	- 0.3 ± 3.8mm	
Mandible To Maxilla				
4.	Effective maxillary length (Co-A)			
5.	Effective mandibular length (Co-Gn)			
6.	Maxillomandibular differential			
7.	Lower anterior facial height (ANS-Me)			
8.	Mandibular plane angle	22.7° ± 4.3°	21.3° ± 3.9°	
9.	Facial axis angle (PTM-Gn and Ba-N)	90° ± 3.2°	90° ± 3.5°	
10.	Upper incisor to point A vertical	5.4 ± 1.7mm	5.3 ± 2.0mm	
11.	Lower incisor protrusion (L1-A-Pog)	2.7 ± 1.7mm	2.3 ± 2.1mm	
Airway				
12.	Upper pharynx	17.4 ± 3.3mm	17.4 ± 4.3mm	
13	Lower pharynx	11.3 ± 3.3mm	13.5 ± 4.3mm	
Soft Tissue Evaluation				
14.	Nasolabial angle	♀ 102° ± 8°	♂ 102° ± 8°	
15.	Cant of upper lip	♀ 13.7 ± 8.2mm	♂ 8.4 ± 7.8mm	

Interpretation:

____

____

____

Attach Lateral Cephalometric tracing here and do COGS Analysis:

COGS Analysis (Hard Tissue) [15, 16, 31, 32]

Sr No.	Measurement	Mean ± SD		Patient's Readings
		Male	Female	
Cranial Base				
1.	Ar-Ptm (Parallel to HP)	37.1mm ± 2.8	32.8mm ± 1.9	
2.	Ptm-Na (Parallel to HP)	52.8mm ± 4.1	50.9mm ± 3.0	
Horizontal Skeletal				
3.	Na-A-Pog	3.9° ± 6.4°	2.6° ± 5.1°	
4.	Na-A (Parallel to HP)	0mm ± 3.7	-2 mm ± 3.6	
5.	Na-B (Parallel to HP)	5.3mm ± 8.5	-6.9mm ± 4.3	
6.	Na-Pog (Parallel to HP)	4.3mm ±8.5	-6.5mm ± 5.1	
Vertical Skeletal And Dental				
7.	Na-ANS (Perp to HP)	54.7mm ± 3.2	50.0mm ± 2.4	
8.	ANS-Gn (Perp to HP)	68.6mm ±3.8	61.3mm ± 3.3	
9.	Na-PNS (Perp to HP)	53.9mm ± 1.7	50.6mm ± 2.2	
10.	MP-HP angle	23° ± 5.9°	24.2° ± 5.0°	
11.	Anterior maxillary dental height (U1-NF) (Perp to NF)	30mm ± 2.1	27.5mm ± 1.7	
12.	Anterior mandibular dental height (L1-MP) (Perp to MP)	45mm ± 2.1	40.8mm ± 1.8	
13.	Posterior maxillary dental height (U6-NF) (Perp to NF)	26.2mm ± 2	23.0mm ± 1.3	
14.	Posterior mandibular dental height (L6-MP) (Perp to MP)	35.8mm ± 2.6	32.1mm ± 1.9	
Maxilla, Mandible				
15.	ANS-PNS	57.7mm ± 2.5	52.6mm ± 3.5	
16.	Ar-Go	52mm ± 4.2	46.8mm ± 2.5	
17.	Go-Pog	83.7mm ± 4.6	74.3mm ± 5.8	
18.	B-Pog (Parallel to MP)	8.9mm ± 1.7	7.2mm ± 1.9	
19.	Ar-Go-Gn	119° ± 6.5°	122° ± 6.9°	
Dental				
20.	OP upper-HP	6.2° ± 5.1°	7.1°±2.5°	
21.	OP lower-HP	-	-	
22.	A-B (Parallel to OP)	-1.1mm ± 2	-0.4mm ± 2.5	
23.	U1-NF	111.1° ± 4.7°	112.5°± 5.3°	
24.	L1-MP	95.9° ± 5.2°	95.9° ± 5.7°	

Interpretation:

____

____

____

Attach Lateral Cephalometric tracing here and do COGS Analysis:

COGS Analysis (Soft Tissue) [15, 16, 31, 32]

Sr No.	Measurement	Mean	± SD	Patient's Readings
	Facial Form			
1.	Facial convexity angle (G-Sn-Pg)	12°	4°	
2.	Maxillary prognathism G-Sn (II HP)	6mm	3mm	
3.	Mandibular prognathism G-Pg (II HP)	0mm	4mm	
4.	Vertical height ratio (G-Sn/Sn-Me)	1:1		
5.	Lower face-throat angle (Sn-Gn-C)	100°	7°	
6.	Lower vertical height- depth ratio (Sn-Gn/C-Gn)	1.2:1		
	Lip Position and Form			
7.	Nasolabial angle (Cm-Sn-Ls)	102°	8°	
8.	Upper lip protrusion (Ls to Sn-Pg’)	3mm	1mm	
9.	Lower lip protrusion (Li to Sn-Pg’)	2mm	1mm	
10.	Mentolabial sulcus (Si to Li-Pg’)	4mm	2mm	
11.	Vertical lip-chin ratio (Sn-Stm$_s$: Stm$_i$- Me’) (PHP)	0.5		
12.	Maxillary incisor exposure (Stm$_s$-1)	2mm	2mm	
13.	Interlabial gap (Stm$_s$-Stm$_i$) (PHP)	2mm	2mm	
	IIHP = Parallel to the horizontal plane PHP = Perpendicular to the horizontal plane			

Interpretation:

____

____

____

Attach Lateral Cephalometric tracing here and do Holdaway Analysis:

Holdaway Analysis (Soft Tissue) [17, 33]

Sr No.	Measurement	Mean ± SD	Patient's Readings
1.	Facial angle	91± 1°	
2.	Upper lip curvature	2.5mm	
3.	Skeletal convexity at point A	-2± 2mm	
4.	H-line angle	7-15°	
5.	Pn-H line		
6.	Upper Sulcus depth	5± 2mm	
7.	Upper lip thickness	15mm	
8.	Upper lip strain		
9.	Li to H line	0 mm (-1 to +2)	
10.	Lower Sulcus depth	5mm	
11.	Chin thickness	10-12mm	
12.	Soft tissue Subnasale (Sn')- H line	5 ±2mm	

Interpretation:

____

____

____

Attach Lateral Cephalometric tracing here and do Powell Analysis:

Powell Analysis [34]

Sr No.	Measurement	Reference Range	Patient's Readings
1.	Nasofrontal angle	115°- 130°	
2.	Nasofacial angle	30°- 40°	
3.	Nasomental angle	120° - 132°	
4.	Nasolabial angle	90° - 110°	
5.	Lip to E-line distance	-2mm	
6.	Mentocervical angle	80° - 95°	

Interpretation:

____

____

____

Attach Lateral Cephalometric tracing here and do Upper Airway Analysis:

Upper Airway Analysis [35]

Sr. No.	Landmarks	Abbreviation
1	Anterior arch of the atlas	AA
2	Intersection of the line drawn at right angles to the pterygoid vertical and 5 mm above the posterior nasal spine (PNS) and the posterior nasopharyngeal wall	Ad
3	Intersection of the line PNS-ba and the posterior nasopharyngeal Wall	ad1
4	Intersection of the line PNS-so and the posterior nasopharyngeal Wall	ad2
5	Basion most posterior limit of the lowest point in the midline on the anterior margin of the foramen magnum	Ba
6	Most posterior points on the inferior margins of the outlines of the bodies of the respective cervical vertebrae	C2 (cv2), C3 (cv3), C4 (cv4)
7	Anteroposterior midpoint on the inferior margin of the body of the second cervical vertebra (axis)	C2c
8	Hormion the most posterior contact point of the vomer with the body of the sphenoid bone;	Ho
9	Hyoidale the most superior point on the anterior surface of the outline of the body of the hyoid bone	Hy
10	Inferior end of the perpendicular from sos to the line that joins PNS to AA	in
11	Most superior point on the tip of the odontoid process	Od
12	Retrognathion; the most inferior point on the posterior surface of the symphsis of the mandible	Rgn
13	Midpoint of the sella-basion line	So
14	Sphenooccipital synchondrosis	Sos
15	Most posterior point on the superior curvature of the tip of the odontoid process	cv2tg

Attach Lateral Cephalometric tracing here and do Upper Airway Analysis:

Linear Measurements for Upper Airway Analysis [35]

Sr. No.	Measurement	Patient's Readings
1	Cervical axis Line od-C5c	
2	Odontoid tangent Line	
3	Pterygoid vertical (PTV)	
4	Anterior cranial base length (S-N),	
5	Posterior cranial base length (ba-S)	
6	Total or effective cranial base length (ba-N)	
7	Length of the palate (PNS-ANS)	
8	Posterior height of the nasal cavity (S-PNS)	
9	Vertical diameter of the choanal openings (ho & PNS)	
10	Floor of the nasopharynx length (AA to PNS)	
11	Total depth of the nasopharynx	
12	Effective length of the maxilla (TMJ to ANS)	
13	Upper anterior facial height (N and ANS)	
14	Distance from so to in	
15	Distance from AA to hy	
16	Distance from hy to rgn	

Angular Measurements for Upper Airway Analysis [35]

Sr. No.	Measurement	Patient's Readings
1	Saddle angle included between the lines joining ba to S and S to N (ba-S-N)	
2	Angle between anterior cranial base & point "A" on maxilla	
3	Angle between the palatal plane (PNS-ANS) and the anterior cranial base (S-N)	
4	Angle of nasopharyngeal depth and the included angle ba-S-PNS	
5	Vertical angle of nasopharynx & angle PNS-ba-S	
6	Roof angle of the nasopharynx and the included angle ba-ho-PNS	
7	Craniocervical angle included between superior extension of the tangent to the posterior surface of the odontoid process and the posterior extension of the line ba-S	

Interpretation:

____

____

____

Superimposition on Longitudinal Cephalogram [15]

Maxillary Superimposition

Mandibular Superimposition

Overall Superimposition

Attach Lateral Cephalometric tracing for Hyoid Triangle Analysis:

Hyoid Triangle Analysis [35]

Landmarks and Planes

Point	Definition
Hyoidale (H point)	The most superior, anterior point on the body of the hyoid bone
Retrognathion (RGn)	The most inferior, posterior point on the mandibular symphysis
C3 point	The most inferior, anterior position on the third cervical vertebrae
Hyoid plane	The plane from H along the long axis of the greater horns of the hyoid bone
Hyoid plane angle	The most superior posterior angle made by the intersection of the hyoid plane with C3-RGn
AA	The most anterior point on the body of the atlas vertebrae
PNS	The tip of the posterior nasal spine

S No.	Measurement	Mean	SD	Finding
1.	H-C3	31.76	± 2.9	
2.	H-RGn	36.83	± 5.83	
3.	C3-RGn	67.2	± 6.6	
4.	H-H	4.80	± 4.64	
5.	Hyoid plane angle	25.63	± 10.59	
6.	AA-PNS	32.91	± 3.66	

Interpretation:

___

___

___

Visualized Treatment Objectives [34]

(Basic VTO with Growth)

(Basic VTO without Growth)

Attach Lateral Cephalometric tracing here and do Predication Tracing for Single Jaw Surgery by overlay method:

Prediction Tracing [14, 34, 36]

(Case 1: Single Jaw Orthognathic Surgery)

Attach Lateral Cephalometric tracing here and do Predication Tracing for Double Jaw Surgery by template method:

Prediction Tracing [14, 34, 36]

(Case 2: Double Jaw Orthognathic Surgery)

Attach PA Cephalometric tracing here and identify land marks on PA Ceph:

Land Marks- Posterior Anterior (PA) Cephalogram

Sr No.	Landmarks	Abbreviations
1.	Antegonion	Ag/AG
2.	Crista galli	Cg/CG
3.	Orbital midpoint	Om
4.	Top nasal septum	tns
5.	Anterior Nasal Spine	Ans/ANS
6.	Mandibular point	m
7.	Menton	Me/M
8.	Latero-orbitale	lo/Lo
9.	Zygomatico frontal lateral suture	lzmf
10.	Zygomatico frontal median suture	mzmf
11.	Condylar	Cd/co
12.	Coronoid	cor
13.	Mastoid	ma
14.	Zygomatic arch	Za/za
15.	Jugale	J
16.	Mental foramen	mf
17.	Lateral piriform aperture	Lpa
18.	Incisor superior frontale	isf
19.	Incisor inferior frontale	iif
20.	Center of the orbit	CO
21.	Eurion	Eu
22.	Gonion	Go
23.	Gnathion	Gn
24.	Frontomalare temporale	Frz
25.	Zygion	Zyg

Attach PA Cephalometric tracing here and do Grummon's Analysis:

Grummon's Analysis [15]

A.	**Horizontal planes**			
1.	Connecting the medial aspects of zygomaticofrontal sutures (Z plane)			
2.	Connecting the centers of the zygomatic arches (ZA);			
3.	One connecting the medial aspects of the Jugal Processes (j);			
4.	Parallel to the Z-plane through Menton.			
B.	**Mid Sagittal Reference Line (MSR)**			
	Measurement	**Right**	**Left**	**Difference**
C.	**Mandibular Morphology Analysis**			
5.	Ag-Me			
6.	Co-Me			
7.	Co-Ag			
8.	Co-Ag-Me			
D.	**Maxillomandibular Comparison**			
9.	Cg- J			
10.	Cg- Ag			
11.	J-MSR			
12.	Ag-MSR			
E.	**Linear Asymmetry Measurement**			
13.	Co-MSR			
14.	NC-MSR			
15.	J-MSR			
16.	Ag-MSR			
F.	**Maxillomandibular Relation**			
17.	J-Buccal cusp			
18.	Ag-Ag			
19.	ANS-Me			
Frontal Vertical Proportion Ratio Analysis				
20.	Upper facial ratio	Cg-ANS: Cg-Me		
21.	Lower facial ratio	ANS-Me: Cg-Me		
22.	Maxillary ratio	ANS-A1: ANS-Me		
23.	Total Maxillary ratio	ANS-A1: Cg-Me		
24.	Mandibular ratio	B1-Me: ANS-Me		
25.	Total Mandibular ratio	B1-Me: Cg-Me		
26.	Maxillomandibular ratio	ANS-A1: B1-Me		

Interpretation:

____

____

____

Attach PA Cephalometric tracing here and do Rickett Analysis (PA):

Rickett Analysis (PA) [15, 37, 38]

Sr No.	Measurement	Mean ± SD	Patient's Readings
	Dental Relations		
1.	Molar relation left (A6-B6)	1.5mm ± 2	
2.	Molar relation right (A6-B6)	1.5mm ± 2	
3.	Inter molar width (B6-B6)	55mm ± 2	
4.	Inter canine width (B3-B3)	22.7mm ± 2	
5.	Denture Midline	0mm ± 1.5	
	Skeletal Relations		
6.	Maxillomandibular width left (ZL-AG)	11mm ± 1.5	
7.	Maxillomandibular width right (ZR-AG)	11mm ± 1.5	
8.	Maxillomandibular midline	0° ± 2°	
9.	Maxillary width (J-J')	61.9mm ± 2	
10.	Mandibular width (AG-GA)	76.1mm ± 2	
	Dental to Skeletal Relations		
11.	Lower molar to jaw left (B6 to J- AG line)	6.3mm ± 1.7	
12.	Lower molar to jaw right (B6 to J-AG line)	6.3mm ± 1.7	
13.	Denture-jaw midlines	0mm ± 1.5	
14.	Occlusal plane tilt	0mm ± 2	
	Jaw to Cranium Relations		
15.	Postural symmetry (Z-AG-ZA left) & (Z-AG-ZA right)	0° ± 2°	
	Internal Structures		
16.	Nasal width	25mm ± 2	
17.	Nasal height (ANS-Z-Z distance)	44.5mm ± 3	
18.	Facial width (ZA-ZA)	116mm ± 3	

Interpretation:

____

____

____

(This page is intentionally left blank)

Growth Prediction

Hand and Wrist Stages

Growth period								
1. PP2 =	2. MP3 =	3. Pisi H1 R =	4. S H2	5. $MP3_{cap}$ R_{cap} $PP1_{cap}$	6. $DP3_u$	7. $PP3_u$	8. $MP3_u$	9. R_u

Stage 4: Just before or beginning of pubertal growth spurt
Stage 5: Peak of pubertal growth spurt
Stage 6: End of pubertal growth spurt
Stage 9: Skeletal growth completed

CVM Stages

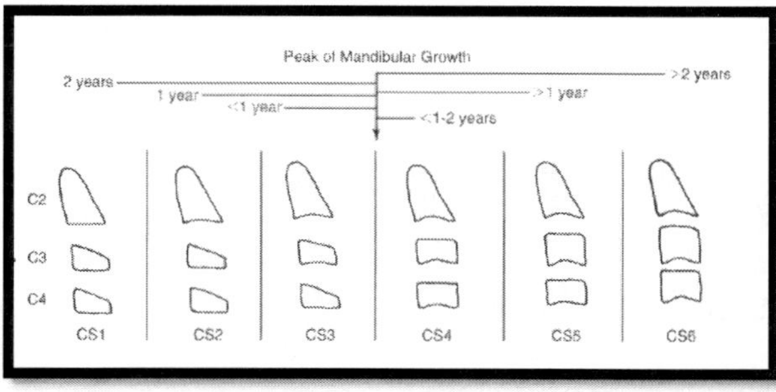

Dental Age Assessment

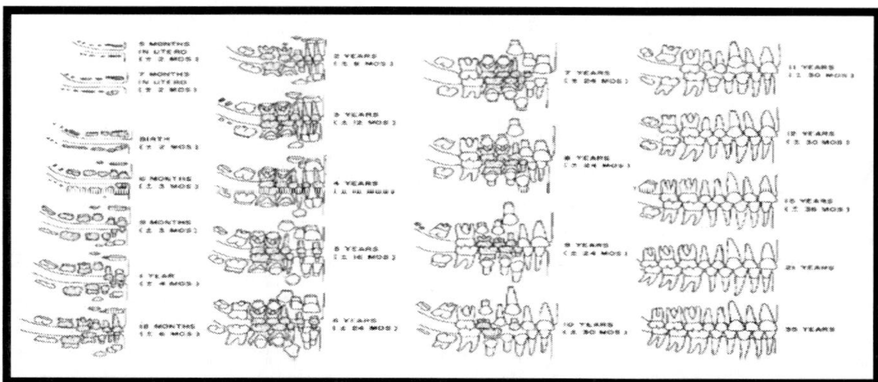

Attach Copy of Hand and Wrist Radiograph, lateral Cephalogram and OPG here:

Case 1

Growth Stage by Hand and Wrist Radiograph

Stage:

___

Significance:

___

Growth Stage by CVM Method

Stage:

___

Significance:

___

Dental Age Assessment by OPG

Chronological age________ Dental Age ___________________

___

Attach Copy of Hand and Wrist Radiograph, lateral Cephalogram and OPG here:

Case 2

Growth Stage by Hand and Wrist Radiograph [27, 39]

Stage:

____

Significance:

____

Growth Stage by CVM Method [27, 40]

Stage:

____

Significance:

____

Dental Age Assessment by OPG [27]

Chronological age________ Dental Age ___________________

____

Cast Analysis

Case 1

Cast Apart

Sr No.	Parameter	Maxilla	Mandible
1.	Arch form		
2.	Arch Symmetry		
3.	Teeth present		
4.	Teeth missing		
5.	Crowding/Spacing (mm)		
6.	Diastema		
7.	Labial/Lingual frenum		
8.	Retroclined		
9.	Proclined		
10.	Buccoversion		
11.	Linguoversion/Palatoversion		
12.	Torsiversion		
13.	Torus Mandibularis		
14.	Any other anomaly		

Cast in Occlusion

		Right	Left
15.	Cuspid relation		
16.	Molar relation		
17.	Incisor Relationship		
18.	Overjet (mm)		
19.	Overbite (mm		
20.	Cross bite		
21.	Dental midline relation		

Case 2

Cast Apart

Sr No.	Parameter	Maxilla	Mandible
1.	Arch form		
2.	Arch Symmetry		
3.	Teeth present		
4.	Teeth missing		
5.	Crowding/Spacing (mm)		
6.	Diastema		
7.	Labial/Lingual frenum		
8.	Retroclined		
9.	Proclined		
10.	Buccoversion		
11.	Linguoversion/Palatoversion		
12.	Torsiversion		
13.	Torus Mandibularis		
14.	Any other anomaly		

Cast in Occlusion

		Right	Left
15.	Cuspid relation		
16.	Molar relation		
17.	Incisor Relationship		
18.	Overjet (mm)		
19.	Overbite (mm		
20.	Cross bite		
21.	Dental midline relation		

SPACE ANALYSIS [27] (DIVIDER METHOD)

Case: 1

Mesiodistal width of upper and lower dentition

	5	4	3	2	1	1	2	3	4	5	Total
Maxilla											
Mandible											

Maxillary arch
Space available: _______
Space required: _______
ALD: _______

Mandibular arch
Space available: _______
Space required: _______
ALD: _______

Diagnosis:

____

____

Case: 2

Mesiodistal width of upper and lower dentition

	5	4	3	2	1	1	2	3	4	5	Total
Maxilla											
Mandible											

Maxillary arch
Space available: ______
Space required: ______
ALD: ______

Mandibular arch
Space available: ______
Space required: ______
ALD: ______

Diagnosis:

____

____

SPACE ANALYSIS [27] (VERNIER CALIPER METHOD)

Case: 1

Mesiodistal width of upper and lower dentition

	5	4	3	2	1	1	2	3	4	5	Total
Maxilla											
Mandible											

Maxillary arch
Space available: _______
Space required: _______
ALD: _______

Mandibular arch
Space available: _______
Space required: _______
ALD: _______

Diagnosis:

____

____

Case: 2

Mesiodistal width of upper and lower dentition

	5	4	3	2	1	1	2	3	4	5	Total
Maxilla											
Mandible											

Maxillary arch
Space available: _______
Space required: _______
ALD: _______

Mandibular arch
Space available: _______
Space required: _______
ALD: _______

Diagnosis:

____

____

Space Analysis [27] (Brass Wire Method)

Case: 1

Mesiodistal width of upper and lower dentition

	5	4	3	2	1	1	2	3	4	5	Total
Maxilla											
Mandible											

Maxillary arch
Space available: _______
Space required: _______
ALD: _______

Mandibular arch
Space available: _______
Space required: _______
ALD: _______

Diagnosis:

____

____

Case: 2

Mesiodistal width of upper and lower dentition

	5	4	3	2	1	1	2	3	4	5	Total
Maxilla											
Mandible											

Maxillary arch
Space available: _______
Space required: _______
ALD: _______

Mandibular arch
Space available: _______
Space required: _______
ALD: _______

Diagnosis:

____

____

Space Analysis [27] (Eye Balling Method)

Case: 1

Maxillary Arch Length Discrepancy (ALD):

Mandibular Arch Length Discrepancy (ALD):

Case: 2

Maxillary Arch Length Discrepancy (ALD):

Mandibular Arch Length Discrepancy (ALD):

ROYAL LONDON SPACE ANALYSIS [41, 42]

Case: 1

Treatment objectives:

1. ______________________________
2. ______________________________
3. ______________________________
4. ______________________________
5. ______________________________

Space requirement:

	Lower arch	Upper arch
Crowding/spacing		
Levelling Curve of Spee		
Arch width change		
Incisor A/P change		
Angulation/inclination change		
Total		

Space creation/utilization:

	Lower arch	Upper arch
Total reduction/enlargement		
Tooth extraction	+	+
Space opening for prosthetic replacement	-	-
Molar distal movement	+	+
Molar mesial movement	-	-
Differential u/l growth (+or-)		

Residue (should be equal to zero):

____

Case: 2

Treatment objectives:

1. ____
2. ____
3. ____
4. ____
5. ____

Space requirement:

	Lower arch	**Upper arch**
Crowding/spacing		
Levelling Curve of Spee		
Arch width change		
Incisor A/P change		
Angulation/inclination change		
Total		

Space creation/utilization:

	Lower arch	**Upper arch**
Total reduction/enlargement		
Tooth extraction	+	+
Space opening for prosthetic replacement	-	-
Molar distal movement	+	+
Molar mesial movement	-	-
Differential u/l growth (+or-)		

Residue (should be equal to zero):

____

Attach Lateral Cephalometric tracing here and do Craniofacial Analysis:

Craniofacial Analysis and Total Space Analysis [35]

Craniofacial Analysis					
Sr No.	**Measurement**	**Range**	**Cephalometric Value**	**Difficulty Factor**	**Difficulty**
1.	FMA	22°-28°		5	
2.	ANB	15°		15	
3.	Z-angle	70°-80°		2	
4.	Occlusal Plane	8°-12°		3	
5.	SNB	78°-82°		5	
6.	Facial height index (PFH=AFH)	0.65-0.75		3	
Craniofacial Difficulty Total:					

Total Space Analysis				
Sr No.	**Measurement**	**Value**	**Difficulty Factor**	**Difficulty**
Anterior				
	Tooth arch discrepancy		1.5	
	Head film discrepancy		1.0	
	Total			
Midarch				
	Tooth arch discrepancy		1.0	
	Curve of Spee		1.0	
	Total			
	Occlusal disharmony (class II or class III)		2.0	
Posterior				
	Tooth arch discrepancy			
	Expected increase (-)			
	Total		0.5	
Space Analysis Difficulty Total:				

Craniofacial Difficulty Total	
Space Analysis Difficulty Total	
Total Difficulty	

Prediction of Prognosis According to Craniofacial Analysis	
Craniofacial difficulty total	**Prediction of prognosis**
over 100	Poor
60-100	Fair
60 and below	Good to Excellent

Interpretation:

___

___

(This page is intentionally left blank)

Mixed Dentition Analysis [27] (Tanaka and Johnston Method)

Mandible

					Total
Mesiodistal width of 2 1 | 1 2 measured on the cast					
	2	1	1	2	
Estimated Mesiodistal width of 5 4 3 | = 1/2 M-D width of 2 1 | 1 2 + 10.5 mm					
Estimated Mesiodistal width of | 3 4 5 = 1/2 M-D width of 2 1 | 1 2 +10.5mm					
Total space required = 2 1 | 1 2 + 543 | 345					

Maxilla

					Total
Mesiodistal width of 2 1 | 1 2 measured on the cast	2	1	1	2	
Estimated Mesiodistal width of 5 4 3 | = 1/2 M-D width of 2 1 | 1 2 +11.0mm					
Estimated Mesiodistal width of | 3 4 5 1/2 M-D width of 2 1 | 1 2 +11.0mm					
Total space required = 2 1 | 1 2 + 5 4 3 | 3 4 5					

	Mandible	Maxilla
Space available		
Space required		
ALD		

Probability Tables for Predicting Sizes of Unerupted Cuspids and Bicuspids

A, Mandibular Bicuspids and Cuspids

21/12 - (%)	19.5	20.0	20.5	21.0	21.5	22.0	22.5	23.0	23.5	24.0	24.5	25.0	25.5
MALES													
95	21.6	21.8	22.0	22.2	22.4	22.6	22.8	23.0	23.2	23.5	23.7	23.9	24.2
85	20.8	21.0	21.2	21.4	21.6	21.9	22.1	22.3	22.5	22.7	23.0	23.2	23.4
75	20.4	20.6	20.8	21.0	21.2	21.4	21.6	21.9	22.1	22.3	22.5	22.8	23.0
65	20.0	20.2	20.4	20.6	20.9	21.1	21.3	21.5	21.8	22.0	22.2	22.4	22.7
50	19.5	19.7	20.0	20.2	20.4	20.6	20.9	21.1	21.3	21.5	21.7	22.0	22.2
35	19.0	19.3	19.5	19.7	20.0	20.2	20.4	20.67	20.9	21.1	21.3	21.5	21.7
25	18.7	18.9	19.1	19.4	19.6	19.8	20.1	20.3	20.5	20.7	21.0	21.2	21.4
15	18.2	18.5	18.7	18.9	19.2	19.4	19.6	19.9	20.1	20.3	20.5	20.7	20.9
5	17.5	17.7	18.0	18.2	18.5	18.7	18.9	19.2	19.4	19.6	19.8	20.0	20.2
FEMALES													
95	20.8	21.0	21.2	21.5	21.7	22.0	22.2	22.5	22.7	23.0	23.3	23.6	23.9
85	20.0	20.3	20.5	20.7	21.0	21.2	21.5	21.8	22.0	22.3	22.6	22.8	23.1
75	19.6	19.8	20.1	20.3	20.6	20.8	21.1	21.3	21.6	21.9	22.1	22.4	22.7
65	19.2	19.5	19.7	20.0	20.2	20.5	20.7	21.0	21.3	21.5	21.8	22.1	22.3
50	18.7	19.0	19.2	19.5	19.8	20.0	20.3	20.5	20.8	21.1	21.3	21.6	21.8
35	18.2	18.5	18.8	19.0	19.3	19.6	19.8	20.1	20.3	20.6	20.9	21.1	21.4
25	17.9	18.1	18.4	18.7	19.0	19.2	19.5	19.7	20.0	20.3	20.5	20.8	21.0
15	17.4	17.7	18.0	18.3	18.5	18.8	19.1	19.3	19.6	19.8	20.1	20.3	20.6
5	16.7	17.0	17.2	17.5	17.8	18.1	18.3	18.6	128.9	·19.1	19.3	19.6	19.8

B, Maxillary Bicuspids and Cuspids

21/12 - (%)	19.5	20.0	20.5	21.0	21.5	22.0	22.5	23.0	23.5	24.0	24.5	25.0	25.5
MALES													
95	21.2	21.4	21.6	21.9	22.1	22.3	22.6	22.8	23.1	23.4	23.6	23.9	24.1
85	20.6	20.9	21.1	21.3	21.6	21.8	22.1	22.3	22.6	22.8	23.1	23.3	23.6
75	20.3	20.5	20.8	21.0	21.3	21.5	21.8	22.0	22.3	22.5	22.8	23.0	23.3
65	20.0	20.3	20.5	20.8	21.0	21.3	21.5	21.8	22.0	22.3	22.5	22.8	23.0
50	19.7	19.9	20.2	20.4	20.7	20.9	21.2	21.5	21.7	22.0	22.2	22.5	22.7
35	19.3	19.6	19.9	20.1	20.4	20.6	20.9	21.1	21.4	21.6	21.9	22.1	22.4
25	19.1	19.3	19.6	19.9	20.1	20.4	20.6	20.9	21.1	21.4	21.6	21.9	22.1
15	18.8	19.0	19.3	19.6	19.8	20.1	20.3	20.6	20.8	21.1	21.3	21.6	21.8
5	18.2	18.5	18.8	19.0	19.3	19.6	19.8	20.1	20.3	20.6	20.8	21.0	21.3
FEMALES													
95	21.4	21.6	21.7	21.8	21.9	22.0	22.2	22.3	22.5	22.6	22.8	22.9	23.1
85	20.8	20.9	21.0	21.1	21.3	21.4	21.5	21.7	21.8	22.0	22.1	22.3	22.4
75	20.4	20.5	20.6	20.8	20.9	21.0	21.2	21.3	21.5	21.6	21.8	21.9	22.1
65	20.1	20.2	20.3	20.5	20.6	20.7	20.9	21.0	21.2	21.3	21.4	21.6	21.7
50	19.6	19.8	19.9	230.1	20.2	20.3	20.5	20.6	20.8	20.9	21.0	21.2	21.3
35	19.2	19.4	19.5	19.7	19.8	19.9	20.1	20.2	20.4	20.5	20.6	20.8	20.9
25	18.9	19.1	19.2	19.4	19.5	19.6	19.8	19.9	20.1	20.2	20.3	20.5	20.6
15	18.5	18.7	18.8	19.0	19.1	19.3	19.4	19.6	19.7	19.8	20.0	20.1	20.2
5	17.8	18.0	18.2	18.3	18.5	18.6	18.8	18.9	19.1	19.2	19.3	19.4	19.5

Mixed Dentition Analysis [43] (Moyer's Prediction Method)

Patient ID: ________________________ **Gender:**________________

Mandible

					Total
Mesiodistal width of 21 | 12 measured on the cast	2	1	1	2	
Mesiodistal width of 543 | as predicted by the table					
Mesiodistal width of | 345 as predicted by the table					
Total space required = 21 | 12 + 543 | 345					

Maxilla

					Total
Mesiodistal width of 21 | 12 measured on the cast	2	1	1	2	
Mesiodistal width of 543 | as predicted by the table					
Mesiodistal width of | 345 as predicted by the table					
Total space required = 21 | 12 + 543 | 345					

	Mandible	**Maxilla**
Space available		
Space required		
ALD		

Attach Lateral Cephalometric tracing here and do Ceph Correction:

MIXED DENTITION ANALYSIS [35] (CEPHALOMETRIC CORRECTION METHOD)

Space Available = ____________ mm

Space Required = I+ 2X+ Ceph. Correction + Curve of Occlusion

	Measurement	Tooth number				Total
I	Sum of mandibular incisors measured on the cast	2	1	1	2	
X'	Radiographic sum of mandibular 5,4,3 of one quadrant	5	4	3		
Y	Sum of mandibular 'e, d, 'c on the cast of the same quadrant	e	d	c		
Y'	Radiographic sum mandibular e, d, c of the same quadrant	e	d	c		
X	**Estimated sum of mandibular 5, 4, 3 =** $\frac{X'Y}{Y'}$					

Ceph Correction= (Proposed FMIA (65°) – Actual FMIA) x 0.8 = mm

Curve of occlusion = $\frac{\text{Right Side Depth + Left Side Depth}}{2}$ + 0.5 = ________mm

Space required = I + 2X + Ceph Correction + Curve of Occlusion = _______mm

Space required =______________mm

Arch Length Discrepancy = mm

BOLTON ANALYSIS [44, 45]

Case: 1

Mesiodistal width of upper and lower dentition

Upper Arch	**6**	**5**	**4**	**3**	**2**	**1**	**1**	**2**	**3**	**4**	**5**	**6**
Lower Arch												
	6	**5**	**4**	**3**	**2**	**1**	**1**	**2**	**3**	**4**	**5**	**6**

Maxillary arch

Sum of 3-3: _______

Sum of 6-6: _______

Mandibular arch

Sum of 3-3: _______

Sum of 6-6: _______

OVERALL RATIO (X)

X = Sum of Mandibular 12 x 100 (Normal 91.3) / Sum of Maxillary 12 = __________X100=__________mm

If X>91.3 (there is mandibular excess)

Desired Sum of Mandibular 12 = Actual Sum of Maxillary 12 x 91.3 / 100 = ___________ / 100 x 91.3=________mm

Amount of overall excessive Mandibular tooth material;

Actual sum of Mandibular 12 – Desired Sum of Mandibular 12 = ___________ = ___________mm

If X < 91.3 (there is maxillary excess)

Desired Sum of Maxillary 12 = Actual Sum of Mandibular 12 x 100 / 91.3 = ___________ / 91.3 x100 = _______mm

Amount of overall Excessive Maxillary tooth material;

Actual sum of Maxillary 12 – Desired Sum of Maxillary 12 = _______________= _____________mm

ANTERIOR RATIO (Y)

Y = Sum of Mandibular 6x100 (Normal77.2) / Sum of Maxillary 6 =______________x 100 =_____________mm

If Y >77.2 (there is mandibular excess)

Desired Sum of Mandibular 6 = Actual Sum of Maxillary 6 x 77.2 / 100 =____________ / 100 x 77.2 =_________mm

Amount of overall excessive Mandibular tooth material:

Actual sum of Mandibular 6 – Desired Sum of Mandibular 6 = _____________= _____________mm

If Y<77.2 (there is maxillary excess)

Desired Sum of Maxillary 6 = Actual Sum of Mandibular 6 x 100 / 77.2 = _____________ / 77.2 x 100=__________mm

Amount of overall Excessive Maxillary tooth material:

Actual sum of Maxillary 6 – Desired Sum of Maxillary 6 = _______________ = _____________mm

Bolton Discrepancy:

Overall: ________________________________

Anterior: _______________________________

Diagnosis:

____

____

____

Quick Check Method:

Overall:__________________________________

Anterior:_________________________________

Interpretation: ____________________________

Treatment Recommendations:

____

____

____

Case: 2

Mesiodistal width of upper and lower dentition

Upper Arch	6	5	4	3	2	1	1	2	3	4	5	6
Lower Arch												
	6	5	4	3	2	1	1	2	3	4	5	6

Maxillary arch
Sum of 3-3: _________
Sum of 6-6: _________

Mandibular arch
Sum of 3-3: _________
Sum of 6-6: _________

OVERALL RATIO (X)

X = Sum of Mandibular 12 x 100 (Normal 91.3) = _________X100=_________mm
Sum of Maxillary 12

If X>91.3 (there is mandibular excess)

Desired Sum of Mandibular 12 = Actual Sum of Maxillary 12 x 91.3 / 100 = _________ / 100 x 91.3=_______mm

Amount of overall excessive Mandibular tooth material;

Actual sum of Mandibular 12 – Desired Sum of Mandibular 12 = ___________ = ___________mm

If X < 91.3 (there is maxillary excess)

Desired Sum of Maxillary 12 = Actual Sum of Mandibular 12 x 100 / 91.3 = _________ / 91.3 x100 = _______mm

Amount of overall Excessive Maxillary tooth material;

Actual sum of Maxillary 12 – Desired Sum of Maxillary 12 = _________= __________mm

ANTERIOR RATIO (Y)

Y = Sum of Mandibular 6x100 (Normal77.2) =_____________x 100 =_____________mm
Sum of Maxillary 6

If Y >77.2 (there is mandibular excess)

Desired Sum of Mandibular 6 = Actual Sum of Maxillary 6 x 77.2 / 100 =___________ / 100 x 77.2 =________mm

Amount of overall excessive Mandibular tooth material:

Actual sum of Mandibular 6 – Desired Sum of Mandibular 6 = _____________= ____________mm

If Y<77.2 (there is maxillary excess)

Desired Sum of Maxillary 6 = Actual Sum of Mandibular 6 x 100 / 77.2 = ___________ / 77.2 x 100=_________mm

Amount of overall Excessive Maxillary tooth material:

Actual sum of Maxillary 6 – Desired Sum of Maxillary 6 = ______________ = ____________mm

Bolton Discrepancy:

Overall: ________________________________

Anterior: _______________________________

Diagnosis:

____

____

____

Quick Check Method:

Overall: ____

Anterior: ____

Interpretation:

____

____

____

Treatment Recommendations:

____

____

____

ABO Discrepancy Index (DI) [46]

Table for Reference

ABO DISCREPANCY INDEX

TOTAL D.I SCORE

OVERJET

≥ 0 to < 1 mm (edge-to-edge)	= 1 pt
≥ 1 to ≤ 3 mm	= 0 pts
> 3 to ≤ 5 mm	= 2 pts
> 5 to ≤ 7 mm	= 3 pts
> 7 to ≤ 9 mm	= 4 pts
> 9 mm	= 5 pts
Negative Overjet (x-bite): 1 pt per mm per tooth	= ____pts
Total	☐

OVERBITE

> 1 to ≤ 3 mm	= 0 pts
> 3 to ≤ 5 mm	= 2 pts
> 5 to ≤ 7 mm	= 3 pts
Impinging (100%)	= 5 pts
Total	☐

ANTERIOR OPEN BITE

0 mm (edge-to-edge), 1 pt per tooth	= ____pts
then 1 pt per mm per tooth	= ____pts
Total	☐

LATERAL OPEN BITE

≥ 0.5 mm, 2 pts per mm per tooth	
Total	☐

CROWDING (only one arch)

≥ 0 to ≤1 mm	= 0 pts
> 1 to ≤3 mm	= 1 pts
> 3 to ≤5 mm	= 2 pts
> 5 to ≤7 mm	= 4 pts
> 7 mm	= 7 pts
Total	☐

OCCLUSAL RELATIONSHIP

Class I to End On	= 0 pts		
End-to-End Class II or III	= 2 pts	per side	____pts
Full Class II or III	= 4 pts	per side	____pts
Beyond Class II or III	= 1 pts		____pts
Total			☐

For mm measures, round up to the next full mm.
Examiners will verify measurements in each category.

LINGUAL POSTERIOR X-BITE

> 0 mm, 1 pt per tooth — Total ☐

BUCCAL POSTERIOR X-BITE

> 0 mm, 2 pts per tooth — Total ☐

CEPHALOMETRICS (See Instructions)

ANB ≥ 6° or ≤ -2°	@4pts	= ____
Each full degree > 6°	____x 1 pt	= ____
Each full degree < 2°	____x 1 pt	= ____
SN-MP		
≥ 38°	@2pts	= ____
Each full degree < 38°	____x 2 pt	= ____
≥ 26°	@1pts	= ____
Each full degree < 26°	____x 1 pt	= ____
$\overline{1}$ to MP ≥ 99°	@1pts	= ____
Each full degree > 99°	____x 1 pt	= ____
Total		☐

OTHER (See Instructions)

Supernumerary teeth	____x 1 pt	= ____
Ankylosis of Permanent teeth	____x 2 pts	= ____
Anomalous morphology	____x 2 pts	= ____
Impaction (except 3rd molars)	____x 2 pts	= ____
Midline discrepancy (≥3 mm)	@ 2 pts	= ____
Missing teeth (except 3rd molars)	____x 1 pts	= ____
Missing teeth, congenital	____x 2 pts	= ____
Spacing (4 or more, per arch)	____x 2 pts	= ____
Spacing (mx cent diastema ≥ 2 mm)	____@ 2 pts	= ____
Tooth transposition	____x 2 pts	= ____
Skeletal asymmetry (nonsurgical tx)	@ 3 pts	= ____
Addl. treatment complexities	____x 2 pts	= ____

Identify:

☐

Total Other ☐

Patients' Name _______________

Parameter	Value	Points
Total		

The American Board of Orthodontics Grading System for Dental Casts and Panoramic Radiographs [47]

Table for Reference

Reference - ABO Cast/Radiograph Evaluation See <u>Grading System for Casts-Radiographs</u> for entire discussion	
ALIGNMENT/ROTATIONS 0.5 - 1 mm = 1 for each tooth $>$ 1 mm = 2 for each tooth	**OCCLUSAL CONTACTS** 0 mm = satisfactory $\le$ 1 mm = 1 (for each posterior $>$ 1 mm = 2 tooth out of contact) ** Do **not** score diminutive distolingual cusps of the maxillary 1st and 2nd molars, nor lingual cusps of the mandibular first premolars. **<u>Maximum of 2 points per tooth</u>**.
MARGINAL RIDGES 0.5 - 1 mm = 1 (for each interproximal contact $>$ 1 mm = 2 between posterior teeth) ** Do **not** include the canine-premolar contact. Do **not** include the distal of lower 1st premolar.	**OCCLUSAL RELATIONSHIP** $<$ 1 mm = satisfactory 1 - 2 mm = 1 (for each maxillary **tooth** from the $>$ 2 mm = 2 the canines to the 2nd molars)
BUCCOLINGUAL INCLINATION 0 - 1 mm = satisfactory 1.1 - 2 mm = 1 (for each posterior tooth) $>$ 2 mm = 2 ** Do **not** score the mandibular 1st premolars nor the distal cusps of the second molars.	**INTERPROXIMAL CONTACTS** 0.6 - 1 mm = 1 (for each interproximal $>$ 1 mm = 2 **contact**)
OVERJET Anterior teeth must be contacting. 0 mm = satisfactory $\le$ 1 mm = 1 (for each maxillary $>$ 1 mm = 2 tooth) Transverse posterior teeth: Mandibular buccal cusps are measured to the central fossa of the maxillary teeth.	**ROOT ANGULATION** Parallel = 0 Not parallel = 1 Root contacting adjacent root = 2 (for each **occurrence**) Do **not** score the maxillary and mandibular canines.

Note: Gauge width is 0.5 mm; Gauge Height is 1 mm

Third molars are not scored unless they substitute for the second molars. No tooth is scored more than two points per individual parameter.

The American Board of Orthodontics
Grading System for Dental Casts and Panoramic Radiographs [47]

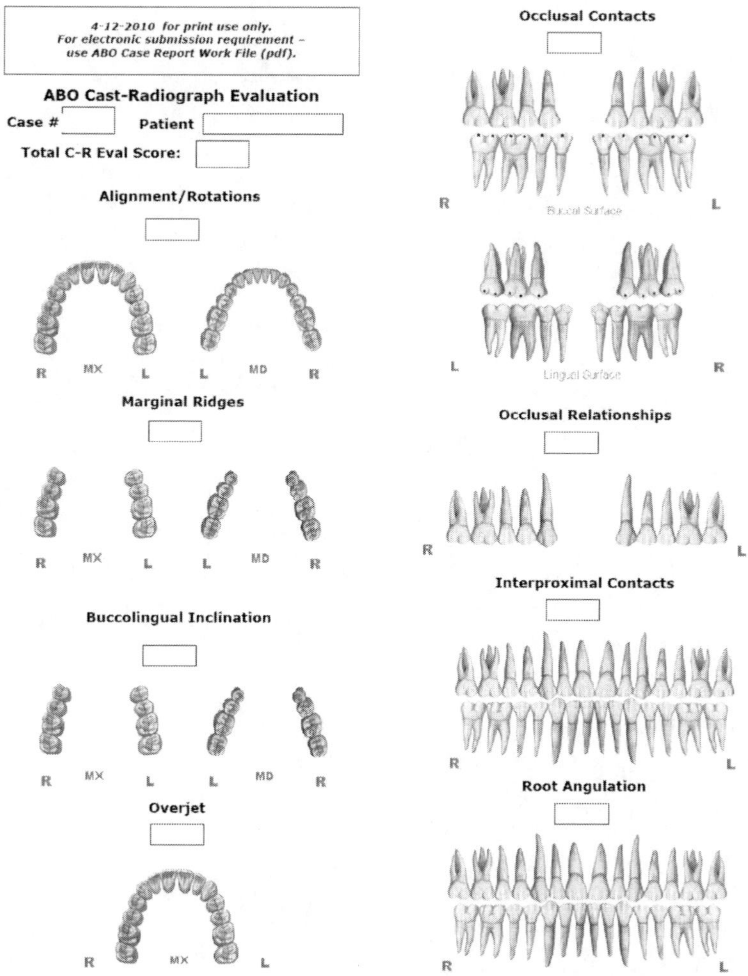
4-12-2010 for print use only.
For electronic submission requirement – use ABO Case Report Work File (pdf).

ABO Cast-Radiograph Evaluation

Case #
Patient
Total C-R Eval Score:

Alignment/Rotations
R MX L L MD R

Marginal Ridges
R MX L L MD R

Buccolingual Inclination
R MX L L MD R

Overjet
R MX L

Occlusal Contacts
R Buccal Surface L
L Lingual Surface R

Occlusal Relationships
R L

Interproximal Contacts
R L

Root Angulation
R L

Instructions: Please score beside each deficient tooth and enter total score for each parameter in the white box. Mark extracted teeth with "X". Second molars should be in occlusion.

Index of Orthodontic Treatment Need (IOTN) [14]

Aesthetic Component

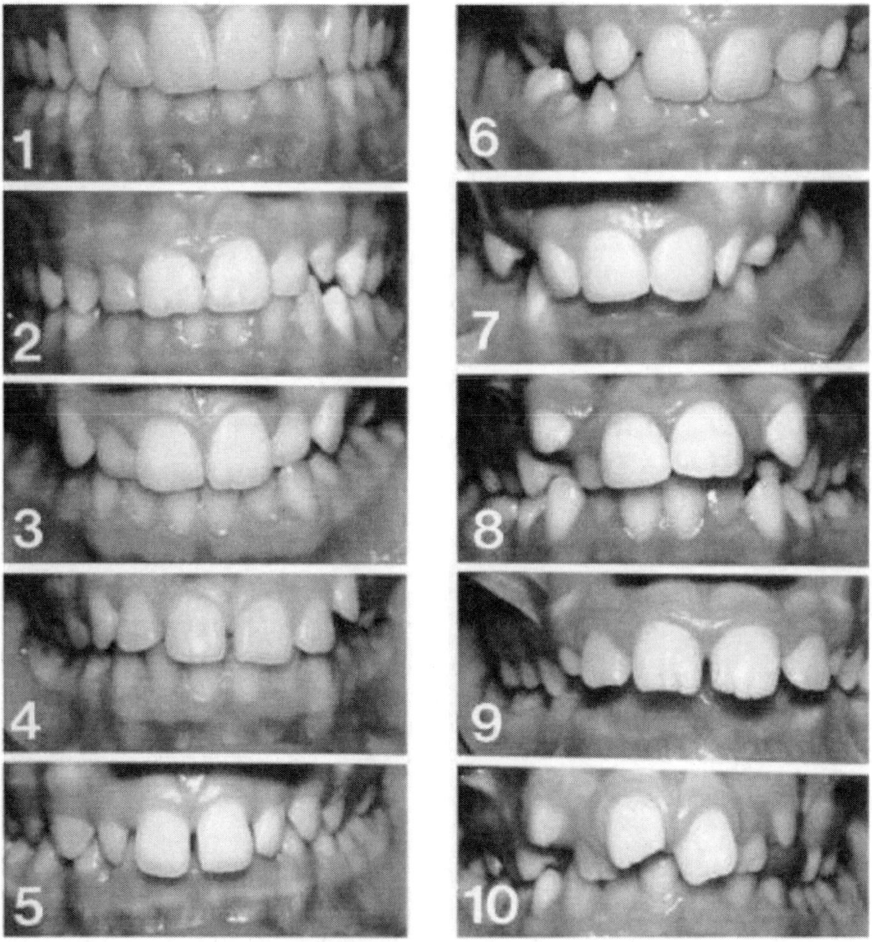

Dental Health Component

DHC	
Grade 5 (Severe)	Defects of cleft lip and/or palate.
	Increased overjet greater than 9 mm.
	Reverse overjet greater than 3.5 mm with reported masticatory or speech difficulties.
Grade 4 (Need)	Impeded eruption of teeth (with the exception of third molars) due to crowding, displacement, the presence of supernumerary teeth, retained primary
	teeth, and any other pathological cause.
	Extensive hypodontia with restorative implication (more than one tooth missing in any quadrant) requiring pre-restorative orthodontics.
Grade 3 (Borderline)	
	Increased overjet greater than 6 mm but less than or equal to 9 mm.
	Reverse overjet greater than 3.5 mm with no reported masticatory or speech difficulties.
Grade 2 (Slight)	Reverse overjet greater than 1 mm but less than or equal to 3.5 mm with reported masticatory or speech difficulties.
Grade 1 (None)	Anterior or posterior crossbites with greater than 2 mm displacement between retruded contact position and intercuspal position.
	Posterior lingual crossbites with no occlusal contact in one or both buccal segments.
	Severe displacement or teeth greater than 4 mm.
	Extreme lateral or anterior open bite greater than 4 mm.
	Increased and complete overbite causing notable indentation on the palate or labial gingivae.
	Patient referred by colleague for collaborative care, for example, periodontal, restorative, or TMJ considerations.
	Less extensive hypodontia requiring pre-restorative orthodontics or orthodontic space closure to obviate the need for a prosthesis (not more than one tooth missing in any quadrant).
	Increased overjet greater than 3.5 mm but less than or equal to 6 mm with incompetent lips at rest.
	Reverse overjet greater than 1 mm but less than or equal to 3.5 mm.
	Increased and complete overbite with gingival contact but without indentations or signs of trauma.
	Anterior or posterior crossbites with less than or equal to 2 mm but greater than 1 mm displacement between retruded contact position and intercuspal position.
	Moderate lateral or anterior open bite greater than 2 mm but less than or equal to 4 mm.
	Moderate displacement of teeth greater than 2 mm but less than or equal to 4 mm.
	Increased overjet greater than 3.5 mm but less than or equal to 6 mm with competent lips at rest.
	Reverse overjet greater than 0 mm but less than or equal to 1 mm.
	Increased overbite greater than 3.5 mm with no gingival contact.
	Anterior or posterior crossbites with less than or equal to 1 mm displacement between retruded contact position and intercuspal position.
	Small lateral or anterior open bites greater than 1 mm but less than or equal to 2 mm.
	Pre-normal or post-normal occlusions with no other anomalies.
	Mild displacement of teeth greater than 1 mm but less than or equal to 2 mm.
	Other variation in occlusion including displacement less than or equal to 1 mm.

Case No______

Aesthetic Component Score_______________________________

Dental Health Component Score___________________________

Need of Treatment_______________________________________

PAR Index

PAR SCORING MATRIX

CASE NUMBER	Pre-treatment										
PAR COMPONENTS	RIGHT								LEFT	WEIGHTED TOTAL	
Upper anterior segments	3-2		2-1		1-1		1-2		2-3		X1	
Lower anterior segments	3-2		2-1		1-1		1-2		2-3		X1	
Buccal occlusion	Antero-posterior			Right			Left			X1	
	Transverse			Right			Left			X1	
	Vertical			Right			Left			X1	
Overjet	Positive					Negative				X6	
Overbite	Overbite					Openbite				X2	
Centre line										X4	
								TOTAL			

CASE NUMBER	Post-treatment										
PAR COMPONENTS	RIGHT								LEFT	WEIGHTED TOTAL	
Upper anterior segments	3-2		2-1		1-1		1-2		2-3		X1	
Lower anterior segments	3-2		2-1		1-1		1-2		2-3		X1	
Buccal occlusion	Antero-posterior			Right			Left			X1	
	Transverse			Right			Left			X1	
	Vertical			Right			Left			X1	
Overjet	Positive					Negative				X6	
Overbite	Overbite					Openbite				X2	
Centre line										X4	
								TOTAL			

PAR SCORE IMPROVEMENT			
Change in PAR Score		Greatly Improved	
% change in PAR score		Improved	
		Worse or No different	

Index of Complexity Outcome and Need (ICON)

A. Icon Scoring Method

Component	Score 0	1	2	3	4	5	Weight
1 Aesthetic assessment	Score 1 to 10						7
2 Upper arch crowding	<2 mm	2.1 to 5 mm	5.1 to 9 mm	9.1 to 13 mm	13.1 to 17 mm	> 17 mm	5
Upper spacing	<2 mm	2.1 to 5 mm	5.1 to 9 mm	>9 mm		Impacted teeth	5
3 Crossbite	No crossbite	crossbite present					5
4 Incisor open bite	Edge to edge	<1 mm	1.1 to 2 mm	2.1 to 4 mm	>4 mm		4
Incisor overbite	<1/3 lower incisor coverage	1/3 to 2/3 coverage	2/3 up to fully covered	Fully covered			4
5 Buccal segment antero-posterior	Cusp to embrasure only Class I, II or III	Any cusp relation up to but not including cusp to cusp	Cusp to cusp				3

1 is judged using IOTN Aesthetic component
2 highest trait judged, either crowding or spacing
4 highest trait judged, either open bite or overbite

Case No______

Pre-treatment

ICON Grade ____________________________________

Need of Treatment________________________________

Post-treatment

ICON Grade ____________________________________

Improvement Grades______________________________

MODULE II

Landmarks of 3D Cephalometry

Sr No.	Hard Tissue Landmark	Abbreviation
1.	Porion	Po_r - Po_l
2.	Orbitale	Or_r - Or_l
3.	Anterior nasal spine	ANS
4.	Posterior nasal spine	PNS
5.	Posterior Maxillary Point:	PMP_r – PMP_l
6.	Upper Incisor	UI_r – UI_l
7.	Lower Incisor	LI_r – LI_l
8.	Upper Molar cusp	$UMcusp_r$ – $UMcusp_l$
9.	Lower Molar Cusp	$LMcusp_r$ – $LMcusp_l$
10.	Menton	Men
11.	Gonion	Go_r – Go_l
12.	Frontozygomatic Point	Fz_r – Fz_l
13.	Zygion	Zy_r – Zy_l
14.	A-Point	A
15.	B-Point	B
16.	Pogonion	Pog
17.	Basion	Ba
18.	Condylion	Co_r – Co_l

Additional 3D Cephalometric Hard Tissue Landmarks

The following list shows some other conventional cephalometric landmarks described in the literature that could be used in 3-D cephalometry.

- Antegonion
- Articulare according to Bjork
- Articulare according to Bolton
- Bolton point
- Bregma
- Coronoid process
- Dacryon
- Frontomaxillary nasal suture
- Frontotemporale
- Glabella
- Gnathion
- Infradentale
- Inferior zygoma
- O-Point
- Opisthion
- Prosthion
- Sellion according to A.M. Schwarz
- Sphenoethmoidal suture
- Spheno-occipital synchondrosis
- Staphylion Supradentale
- Temporale
- Vertex
- Zygion

Landmarks of 3D Cephalometry

Sr No.	Soft Tissue Landmarks	Abbreviation
1.	Glabella	g
2.	Soft tissue nasion	n
3.	Sellion (subnasion)	se
4.	Endocanthion	en_r, en_l
5.	Exocanthion	ex_r, ex_l
6.	Maxillofrontale	mf_r,mf_l
7.	Soft tissue orbitale	or_r - or_l
8.	Orbitale superius	os_r, os_l
9.	Zygion	zy_r, zy_l
10.	Tragion	t_r, t_l
11.	Pronasale	prn
12.	Subnasale	sn_r', sn_l'
13.	Alare	al_r, al_l
14.	Alar curvature point	ac_r, ac_l
15.	Nostril top point	nt_r, nt_l
16.	Columella constructed point	c''
17.	Nostril base point	nb_r, nb_l
18.	Subspinale	ss
19.	Labiale (or labrale) superius	ls
20.	Crista philtri	cph_r, cph_l
21.	Stomion	sto
22.	Cheilion	ch_r, ch_l
23.	Labiale (or labrale) inferius	li
24.	Soft tissue gonion	go_r, go_l
25.	Sublabiale	sl
26.	Soft tissue pogonion	pg
27.	Soft tissue gnathion	gn

Planes of 3D Cephalometry

Sr No.	Name	Abbreviation
1.	Frankfort horizontal Plane	FH-Pl
2.	Maxillary Plane	Mx-Pl
3.	Occlusal Plane	Occ-Pl
4.	Mandibular Plane	Md-Pl
5.	Facial Mid Plane Virtual	
6.	Supraorbital margin plane	
7.	Midsagittal Plane	
8.	Coronal Plane	
9.	Mid maxillary plane	
10.	Ramal Plane	
11.	Mid mandibular Plane	
12.	Facial Mid Plane	

Paste a print out here after 3D Cephalometric tracing on the software:

3D Cephalometric Analysis [48-53]

Sr No.	Measurement	Readings		Patient's Readings
		Male	**Female**	
1.	**SNA angle (°)**	82.5 ± 3.2	81.6 ± 3.2	
2.	**SNB angle (°)**	80.4 ± 3.1	79.2 ± 3.0	
3.	**ANB angle (°)**	2.1 ± 1.8	2.5 ± 1.8	
4.	**Sum (°)**	390.3 ± 5.5	393.2 ± 5.2	
5.	**Mn plane angle (°)**	30.3 ± 5.5	33.4 ± 5.1	
6.	**Upper lip (mm)**	- 0.7 ± 2.2	0.9 ± 2.2	
7.	**Lower lip (mm)**	0.5 ± 2.3	0.6 ± 2.3	
8.	**U1 to SN (°)**	106.± 3 6	106.9 ± 6.0	
9.	**IMPA (°)**	96.6 ± 6.6	95.9 ± 6.4	
10.	**Zygoma**			
	Facial index	87.1 ± 4.7	88.8 ± 5.9	
	Midfacial length			
	Right	125.9 ± 8.8	129.0 ± 8.5	
	Left	126.0 ± 7.7	130.6 ± 6.8	
	Difference	0.1 ± 2.9	0.1 ± 2.7	
11.	**Maxilla**			
	canting (°)	0.5 ± 1.3	0.4 ± 1.2	
	rotation (°)	0.1 ± 1.6	- 0.6 ± 0.9	
	divergence (°)	- 6.7 ± 4.8	- 21.3 ± 3.6	
12.	**Mandible**			
	canting (°)	0.0 ± 1.2	0.3 ± 1.5.	
	rotation (°)	-1.1 ± 1.8	- 0.8 1.4	
	divergence (°)	27.4 ± 4.2	30.9 ± 5.8	

Paste a case after 3D Predication tracing and Soft Tissue Morphing using View Box, etc. to visualize treatment effects:

Viewbox 4 Cephalometric Software [54]

	Mandibular measurements			
13.	**Body length (mm)**			
	Right	94.7 ± 5.2	88.9 ± 3.9	
	Left	96.8 ± 5.9	91.5 ± 2.8	
	Difference	- 1.3 ± 2.4	- 2.8 ± 2.6	
14.	**Gonial angle** (°)			
	Right	118.9 ± 4.4	125.0 ± 4.3	
	Left	118.6 ± 5.4	123.6 ± 5.3	
	Difference	0.6 ± 2.0	1.4 ± 1.9	
15.	**Ramus height (mm)**			
	Right	60.7 ± 6.4	51.5 ± 2.7	
	Left	60.0 ± 7.2	50.5 ± 4.2	
	Difference	1.0 ± 4.6	1.9 ± 4.9	
16.	**Internal Ramal inclination** (°)			
	Right	91.9 ± 4.3	90.3 ± 5.3	
	Left	91.9 ± 5.1	91.4 ± 4.6	
	Difference	0.0 ± 1.4	- 1.1 ± 1.4	
17.	**External Ramal inclination** (°)			
	Right	80.6 ± 3.3	82.2 ± 4.3	
	Left	81.0 ± 2.6	81.4 ± 3.6	
	Difference	- 0.4 ± 1.8	0.8 2.0	
18.	**Lateral Ramal inclination** (°)			
	Right	86.0 ± 2.5	83.4 ± 3.2	
	Left	85.7 ± 2.5	85.0 ± 3.6	
	Difference	0.2 ± 1.8	- 1.4 ± 1.6	
19.	**Chin prominence (mm)**			
	Abs	4.6 ± 0.8	4.0 ± 0.6	
	Rel.	4.7 ± 0.8	4.4 ± 0.6	
	Mn-face width	1.0 ± 0.1	1.0 ± 0.0	
20.	**Facial convexity Bc:A:B:Pog**			
	Right	0.0:0.1:0.1 ± 0.2:0.4:0.4 1	0.1:0.2:0.2 ± 0.1:0.3:0.3	
	Left	0.0:0.1:0.1 ±0.2:0.4:0.4	0.1:0.2:0.2± 0.1:0.3:0.3	

Interpretation:

____

____

____

REFERENCES

[1] Mahmood, A; Nazir, R. A Structured Programme for Post Graduate Training in Orthodontics. *Pak Orthod J.*, 2014, 6(2), 87-108.

[2] Anderson, LW; et al. *A Taxonomy for Learning, Teaching, and Assessing: A revision of Bloom's Taxonomy of Educational Objectives*. New York: Pearson, Allyn & Bacon, 2001.

[3] Giles, JA. Peer assisted learning, take control of your own teaching and learning. *Student BMJ.*, 2009, 17, b2498.

[4] Dental curriculum in the intercollegiate curriculum programme [homepage on the internet] (cited 2015, Feb 15). Available from: https://www.iscp.ac.uk/dental/wbas.aspx.

[5] Kumar, V; Gadbury-Amyot, CC. A case-based and team-based learning model in oral and maxillofacial radiology. *J Dent Educ.*, 2012, 76 (3), 330-7.

[6] Singh, T; Anshu. *Principles of Assessment in Medical Education*. New Delhi: Jaypee, 2012, 59.

[7] Wilkinson, TJ. Assessment of clinical performance. Gathering evidence. *Intern Med J.*, 2007, 37, 631–6.

[8] General Medical Council. *Workplace-Based Assessment: A Guideline for implementation*. London: GMC, 2010.

[9] Jacobson, A; Jacobson, RL. editors. *Radiographic cephalometry: from basics to 3-D imaging*. Quintessence Pub., 2006.

[10] Athanasiou, AE. editor. *Orthodontic cephalometry*. Mosby-Wolfe; 1995.

[11] Rakosi, T. *An atlas and manual of cephalometric radiography*. Lea & Febiger, 1982.

[12] Mitchell, L. *An introduction to orthodontics*. Oxford University Press. 3rd edition.

[13] Atack, NE; Turner, SR; Thomas, P; Nattrass, C; Sandy, JR. *Postgraduate Notes in Orthodontics: MSc/MOrth programme;* 8th ed. University of Bristol, 2019.

[14] Proffit, WR; White, RP; Sarver, DM. *Contemporary treatment of dentofacial deformity*. Mosby, 2003.

[15] Athanasiou, AE. *Orthodontic cephalometry*. London: Mosby-Wolfe.6th edition, 1995.

[16] Malcom, EM; Cangialosi, TJ. *A guide to cephamlometrics*.

[17] Jacobson, A; Jacobson, RL. editors. *Radiographic cephalometry: from basics to 3-D imaging*. Quintessence Pub., 2006.

[18] Jacobson, A. The "Wits" appraisal of jaw disharmony. *Am J Orthodont*., 1975, 1, 67(2), 125-38.

[19] Jacobson, A. Application of the" Wits" appraisal. *Am J Orthodont*., 1976, 70(2), 179-89.

[20] Wylie, WL. The assessment of anteroposterior dysplasia. *The Angle Orthodont*., 1947, 17(3), 97-109.

[21] Wylie, WL; Johnson, EL. Rapid evaluation of facial dysplasia in the vertical plane. *The Angle Orthodont*., 1952, 22(3), 165-82.

[22] Steiner, CC. Cephalometrics for you and me. *Am J Orthod*., 1953, 39, 729-55.

[23] Steiner, CC. Cephalometrics in clinical practice. *Angle Orthod*., 1959, 29, 8-29.

[24] Tweed, CH. The Frankfort – mandibular plane angle in orthodontic diagnosis, classification, treatment planning, and prognosis. *Am J Orthod*., 1946, 32, 175-230.

[25] Tweed, CH. Evolutionary trends in orthodontics, past, present, and future. *Am J Orthod.*, 1953, 39, 81-94.

[26] Tweed, CH. The Frankfort – mandibular incisor angle (FMIA) in orthodontic diagnosis, treatment planning and prognosis. *Angle Orthod.*, 1954, 24, 121-69.

[27] Proffit, WR. *Contemporary orthodontics.* St. Louis, Mo: Mosby Elsevier., 2019.

[28] Sassouni, V. A Roentgenographic cephalometric analysis of cephalo-facio-dental relationships. *Am J Orthod.*, 1955, 41, 735-64.

[29] Sassouni, V. A classification of skeletal facial types. *Am J Orthod.*, 1969, 55, 109-23.

[30] McNamara, JA; Brudon, WL. *Orthodontic and orthopaedic treatment in the mixed dentition.* Ann Arbor, MI: Needham Press. 1995.

[31] Burstone, CJ; James, RB; Legan, H; Murphy, GA; Norton, LA. Cephalometrics for orthognathic surgery. *J Oral Surg.*, 1978, 36(4), 269-77.

[32] Legan, HL; Burstone, CJ. Soft tissue cephalometric analysis for orthognathic surgery. *J Oral Surg.*, 1980, 38, 744–51.

[33] Holdaway, RA. A soft-tissue cephalometric analysis and its use in orthodontic treatment planning. Part I. *Am J Orthod.*, 1983, 84(1), 1–28.

[34] Gregoret, J. *Orthodontics and orthognathic surgery: Diagnosis and planning.* Barcelona: Espaxs., 2003.

[35] Graber, TM; Vanarsdall, RL; Vig, KW. *Orthodontics, current principles and techniques.* St Louis. The upper airway and Craniofacial Morphology. 4th edition, Chapter 4, p. 130.

[36] Reyneke, JP. *Essentials of orthognathic surgery.* Quintessence Publishing., 2 ed, 2010.

[37] Ricketts, RM. The sources of computerized In: Ricketts RM, Bench RW (eds). *Manual of Advanced Orthodontics Seminar*, 1970.

[38] Ricketts, RM. The value of Cephalometrics. and computerized technology. *Am J Orthod.*, 1972, 42, 179-99.

[39] Rakosi, T; Jonas, I; Graber, TM. *Orthodontic diagnosis*. Stuttgart: G. Thieme Medical Publishers, 1993.

[40] McNamara, JA; Jr. Franchi, L. The cervical vertebral maturation method: A user's guide. *Angle Orthod.*, 2018, 88(2), 133-143.

[41] Kirschen, RH; O'higgins, EA; Lee, RT. The Royal London Space Planning: an integration of space analysis and treatment planning: Part I: Assessing the space required to meet treatment objectives. *Am J Orthod Dentofacial Orthop.*, 2000, 118(4), 448-55.

[42] Kirschen, RH; O'Higgins, EA; Lee, RT. The Royal London Space Planning: an integration of space analysis and treatment planning: Part II: The effect of other treatment procedures on space. *Am J Orthod Dentofacial Orthop.*, 2000, 118(4), 456-61.

[43] Moyers, RE. *Handbook of orthodontics*. 4th ed. Chicago: Year Book; 1991, p. 198-201.

[44] Bolton, WA. Disharmony in tooth size and its relation to the analysis and treatment of malocclusion. *Angle Orthodont.*, 1958, 28(3), 113-30.

[45] Bolton, WA. The clinical application of a tooth-size analysis. *Am J of Orthodont.,* 1962, 48(7), 504-29.

[46] Cangialosi, TJ; Riolo, ML; Owens, Jr. SE; Dykhouse, VJ; Moffitt, AH; Grubb, JE; Greco, PM; English, JD; James, RD. The ABO discrepancy index: a measure of case complexity. *Am J Orthod Dentofacial Orthop.*, 2004, Mar 1, 125(3), 270-8.

[47] The American Board of Orthodontics Grading System for Dental Casts and Panoramic Radiographs [Internet] [Revised June 2012] Available from: https://www.americanboardortho.com/media/1191/grading-system-casts-radiographs.pdf.

[48] Bayomea, Park JH; Kook, YH. New three-dimensional cephalometric analyses among adults with a skeletal Class I pattern and normal occlusion. *Korean J Orthod*, 2013, 43(2), 62-73.

[49] Cho, HJ. A three-dimensional cephalometric analysis. *Journal of clinical orthodontics: JCO*, 43(4), 235-52.

[50] Bayome M, Park JH, Kim Y, Kook YA. 3D analysis and clinical applications of CBCT images. *Seminars in Orthodontics.,* 2015, 21(4), pp. 254-262.

[51] Swennen, GR; Schutyser, FA; Hausamen, JE. editors. *Three-dimensional cephalometry: a colour atlas and manual.* Springer Science & Business Media, 2005.

[52] Park, SH; Yu, HS; Kim, KD; Lee, KJ; Baik, HS. A proposal for a new analysis of craniofacial morphology by 3-dimensional computed tomography. *Am J Orthod Dentofacial Orthop.*, 2006, 129(5), 600-e23.

[53] Devanna, R. Two-dimensional to three-dimensional: A new three-dimensional cone-beam computed tomography cephalometric analysis. *J Orthod Res.*, 2015, 3, 30-7.

[54] *Viewbox 4 Cephalometric* Software by dHAL software [Internet] [Revised 2019 Available from: http://www.dhal.com/downloads/viewbox4_manual.pdf.

INDEX

#

1st, 2nd, 3rd order bends, 46, 52
3-D Digitized landmarks identification & Cephalometric, 34

A

ABO Discrepancy Index, 26, 234
ABO Grading, 26, 70, 76, 83
academic, 13
Acceptance of Research paper 1 for publication, 46, 52
adjunctive orthodontics, 46, 49
administrative, 13
adult orthodontics, 46, 48, 49
affective domain, 1
aligners, 72, 73, 74
analysis, 20, 23, 24, 26, 34, 46, 71, 72, 74, 141, 154, 155, 160, 161, 162, 163, 172, 173, 194, 204, 205, 225, 227, 229, 251, 252, 253
anchor bend, 52, 121
anchorage, 27, 28, 29, 31, 39, 117, 131
annexures, x, xiii, 2, 4, 97
anterior positioning appliance, 61
anterior retraction, 58, 67, 121, 127
Appliance systems (Begg, Tip edge, Tweed, Damon, MBT, etc.), 46, 47, 49
Approval of synopsis for Dissertation/Thesis, 52
arch forms, 46, 52
arch lengthening & expansion, 36, 40
article(s), 1, 7, 8, 23, 26, 30, 39, 43, 48, 57, 61, 66, 73, 76, 77, 79
Articulation & fabrication of functional appliance, 36, 43
assessment, x, xiii, xiv, xvii, 1, 2, 3, 4, 11, 15, 16, 20, 25, 28, 33, 36, 42, 46, 51, 53, 56, 60, 64, 69, 72, 75, 78, 82, 85, 87, 97, 98, 99, 100, 101, 102, 103, 104, 106, 107, 109, 110, 112, 114, 116, 118, 120, 122, 124, 126, 128, 130, 132, 134, 136, 138, 139, 209, 211, 213, 249, 250
Auxiliaries, 46, 52, 115, 116, 117, 118

B

ball ended clasp, 20, 26
ball stop(s), 64, 66, 67, 70, 129
band cementation typodont, 34
basic learning, 1
basic life support, 4
bend, 52, 161
Bi-Annual Review Proforma, xvii, 2

bilateral helices, 121
bilateral retraction loops, 127
biomechanics & mechanics, 28, 31
biostatistics, 4, 27, 46, 49
bite corrector, 70
Bite planes (ant/post), 36, 41, 43
bolton analysis, 26, 230
bracket bonding, 28, 110
bracket bonding typodont, 34
bull, 52
burstone arch, 52

C

canine retractor, 20, 26
case based discussion, xvii, 2
cast analysis, 20, 23, 24, 26, 141, 214
CBCT interpretation, 34
C-clasp, 26
cell, 20, 21, 24
Cephalometric Analysis, 26, 76, 245
Cephalometric Correction (SN-FH Correction), 150, 151, 229
Cephalometric Correction Method, 229
checklist, x, xiii, xvii, 2, 17, 26, 34, 43, 52, 61, 70, 76, 83
chin cup, 35, 36, 41, 43
Circumferential Supracrestal Fiberotomy, 123
Class I/II/III Retraction, 121
Cleft Lip & Palate, 55, 56, 58
cleft lip and palate (basic knowledge), 20, 23, 24
Clinical Audit, 63, 64
Clinical Governance, 64, 65
Clip on retainer, 52
Closure of residual spaces, 46
COGS Analysis (Soft Tissue), 132, 145, 157, 179, 180, 181, 182, 183, 185, 243, 246
commencement, 8
communication skills, 4, 27
Comprehensive Case Record(s), 15, 28, 31, 36, 41, 43, 46, 50, 64, 70, 72, 74, 76, 78, 80, 83
comprehensive orthodontics, 15
Craniofacial Analysis, 222, 223
Craniofacial anomalies/ syndromes, 20
crimpable hook, 129
critical incident technique, xvii, 2
curriculum, ix, x, xiii, 1, 7, 249

D

debonded cases, 15, 70, 76, 83
debonding, 15
development of dentition & occlusion, 28, 31
diagnosis, 11, 21, 22, 38, 47, 48, 98, 157, 177, 216, 217, 218, 231, 233, 251
digitized landmarks identification, 76
direct observation of procedural skills, xvii, 2
disciplinary procedures, 78, 79, 80
dissertation writing, 4, 35, 45
distal jet, 66, 70, 131, 132
distraction osteogenesis, 63, 64, 65
disturbances in dental development including impacted teeth, 36, 40
divider method, 216
dolphin imaging 1, 76
double jaw surgery, 200

E

eastman correction, 148, 149
embryology, 20, 24
erverdi plate, 43
essex type, 46, 52
ethics and professionalism, 36
exit examination, 5, 17
extraction vs non-extraction, 46

extra-oral traction, 36, 40

F

face bow record and mounting, 61
face bow recording, 125
face mask, 35, 36, 41, 43
facial asymmetries, 55, 56, 57, 58
feedback, xv, 2, 7, 8, 11, 97, 98, 99, 100, 101, 102, 103, 104, 105, 106, 107, 108, 109, 110, 111, 112, 113, 114, 115, 116, 117, 118, 119, 120, 121, 122, 123, 124, 125, 126, 127, 128, 129, 130, 131, 132, 133, 134, 135, 136, 137, 138, 139
feeding plate, 26
financial record keeping, 77, 78, 79, 80, 83
finger spring, 20, 26
finishing and detailing, 133
fitting molar bands, 107
fixed & removable appliances, 28, 31
fixed retainer, 52
formative, 2, 4
forsus appliance, 38, 43

G

genetics, 19, 20, 21, 24
gingivectomy, 58, 123, 124
gingivoplasty, 58, 123
growth and development, 20, 24
growth predication, 26
growth prediction, 141

H

habit breaking appliance, 28
headgear, 35, 37, 39, 43
History of orthodontics, 46, 47, 49
Holdaway Analysis, 184, 185
Hyoid Triangle Analysis, 195
Hyrax, 36, 43

I

iatrogenic effects of orthodontic treatment, 46, 49
ICON, 26, 241
implants, 36, 38, 40, 113
Impression & Bite registration for functional appliance, 43
Inclined plane, 36, 41, 43
Index of Complexity Outcome and Need (ICON), 26, 241
Index of Orthodontic Treatment Need (IOTN), 26, 238, 241
indexed journals, 12
indices, 27, 28, 29, 31, 141
indirect bonding, 71, 72, 73, 74, 76
instructional strategies, xvii, 1, 3, 7, 16, 20, 28, 36, 46, 56, 64, 72, 78
introduction to computer, 4
intrusion arches, 52

J

Jig, Jones, 70, 131, 132
journal club meetings, 1
journals, 1, 7, 23, 30, 39, 48, 57, 66, 73, 77, 78, 79, 80
Jumper, Jasper, 70

K

kesling setup, 45, 52
knowledge, x, xiv, xvii, 1, 2, 3, 4, 7, 20, 24, 25, 27, 28, 31, 33, 36, 40, 42, 45, 46, 49, 51, 53, 56, 58, 60, 64, 67, 69, 71, 72, 74, 75, 78, 80, 82, 85, 87, 88, 98, 99, 100, 101

L

labial bow, 20, 26
LASERS, 71, 72, 74
lingual orthodontics, 29, 63, 64, 65, 67
lip bumper, 28, 34
Lolly pop, 52
Long Clinical Case, xvii, 2, 85
loops, 46, 52, 67, 96, 119, 127, 128

M

magnets, 63
magnets, 63, 64, 65, 67
malocclusions, 35, 36, 40, 252
management of staff, 78, 79, 80
mandatory, 1, 2, 4, 5, 7, 8, 9, 12, 17, 28, 88, 89, 97, 98, 99, 100, 101, 102, 103, 104, 105, 107, 108, 110, 111, 113, 115, 117, 119, 121, 123, 125, 127, 129, 131, 133, 135, 137, 139
mandatory workshops, 4, 17, 28
mandibular superimposition, 192
MARA, 66, 70
Maxillary Superimposition, 192
McNamara Analysis, 178, 179
MCQs, 2, 3, 20, 25, 28, 33, 36, 42, 46, 51, 53, 56, 60, 64, 69, 72, 75, 77, 78, 79, 82, 85, 93
medical conditions related to dentistry, 20, 22, 24
medical writing, 46, 64, 78, 79
Medicolegal aspects of practice, 64, 65, 67
Mini-Clinical Evaluation Exercise, xvii, 2
mini-implant insertion, 113
Minor Oral surgery (CSF, high frenum, etc.), 56, 57, 58
mixed dentition, 20, 23, 24, 26, 29, 30, 141, 225, 227, 229, 251
mixed dentition analysis, 141
model surgery, 56, 58, 61
model trimming, 20, 23, 24, 26
modified sassouni analysis, 176, 177
Module I, x, 4, 5, 15, 16, 17, 25, 26, 53, 85, 89, 97, 98, 99, 100, 102, 103, 104, 105, 107, 108, 110, 111, 113, 115, 117, 119, 141, 242
molecular biology, 19, 20, 24
mouth guard, 28, 34
Mulligan Mechanics, 52
multiple choice questions, 2

N

nitinol expander, 36, 43

O

obstructive sleep apnea, 64, 65, 67
occlusion, 27, 29, 36, 37, 40, 48, 57, 138, 214, 215, 229, 237, 252
opus, 52
oral physiology, 36, 40
oral screen, 28, 34
orthodontic diagnosis
  (development of problem list), 20, 21, 22, 23, 24, 28, 30, 31, 38, 252
orthodontic diagnosis & treatment planning, 28, 31
orthodontic diagnosis (development of problem list), 19, 20, 24, 27, 250, 251
orthodontic materials, 27, 28, 30, 31
orthodontic research, 46, 56
orthodontic research for dissertation writing, 46
Orthodontic treatment Phase II, 46, 47, 48, 49
Orthodontic treatment Phase III (finishing), 46, 48
orthognathic surgery, 56, 57, 58
orthopaedics, 36, 37, 40, 65
out bend, 52

over jet correction, 46, 47
overall superimposition, 193
overbite correction, 46, 47
overlay, 198

P

PAR Index, 26, 240
Past FCPS papers, 78
patient behaviour, 20, 21, 24
patient progress proforma, xiv, xvii, 2, 101
pendulum appliance, 70
periodontal problems, 46, 49
photography, 20, 23, 24, 26, 104
piggyback wire, 117
placement of arch wire, 115
Posterior Anterior (PA) Cephalogram, 203
postgraduate, ix, xiii, xiv, 1, 3
postgraduate orthodontics, 1
Powell Analysis, 186, 187
Prediction tracing, 56, 57, 58, 61
Presentations, 1, 7
Preventive & interceptive orthodontics, 28, 31
Proforma, xiv, 2, 3, 4, 7, 8, 11, 87
programme, x, xiii, xiv, xv, 1, 3, 249, 250
psychology & motivation, 20
publications, 12

Q

Quad helix, 36, 43
question(s), iv, xvii, 2, 3, 38, 105

R

radiography, 30, 250
Radiology and radiography, 28
reassessed, 4
Research Methodology, 4, 27, 49
Retainers, 46, 50, 52
Retention, 45, 46, 49, 80, 111, 137, 138
Retention & relapse, 46, 49
reverse helical, 52
Rickett Analysis, 206, 207
Rotating springs, 52
Royal London space, 26
Royal London Space Analysis, 220

S

Sabbagh Universal Spring, 70
Sassouni Analysis, 174, 175
Segmental Canine Retraction, 119
Self-ligating brackets, 71, 72, 73, 74
Short Answer Questions, 2
Short Clinical Case, xviii, 2
Single Jaw Surgery, 198
skills and attitudes, 1
Smile aesthetics, 36, 40
Soldering/welding, 28, 34
Space Analysis, 26, 141, 216, 217, 218, 219, 223, 252
Space Analysis (Brass Wire Method), 141, 218, 252
Space Analysis (Eye Balling Method), 26, 216, 217, 218, 219, 223
space maintainer, 28, 34
stabilization appliance, 61
staff management, 77, 78, 80, 83
steiner analysis, 164, 165
store keeping, 77, 78, 79, 80, 83
structured training program, 3
study topics, 1, 7
succeeding module, 5
summative, 2, 4
Superimposition, 192
Surgical Splint fabrication (Intermediate+ Final), 61
Synopsis Writing, 28

Systemic effects of orthodontic treatment, 56, 57, 58

T

T- spring, 26
Tanaka and Johnston Method, 225
Task Oriented Assessment of Clinical Skills, xviii, 2
Teaching & learning, 36, 40, 46
template methods, 198, 200
theories, 1
TMJ Examination, 28, 31, 45, 46, 48, 49, 105, 106, 191
toe in, 52
toe out, 52
torqueing springs, 52
total space analysis, 223
TPA/Nance button fabrication/Lingual arch, 34
trainees, xiii, 1, 3, 4, 7, 8, 11, 13, 85
Trauma and orthodontics, 56, 57, 58
treatment planning session, 11, 65
tweed analysis, 168, 169
tweed triangle, 170, 171

U

upper airway analysis, 188, 189, 190, 191
utility arch, 52

V

vernier caliper method, 217
view box, 34, 74, 76
visualized treatment objectives, 196
viva, 2, 3, 20, 28, 36, 46, 56, 64, 72, 78

W

w-arch, 36, 43
whip spring, 28, 34
wilson arch, 70
wits appraisal, 152, 153
workplace-based assessment, xviii, 2, 249
wylie analysis, 158, 159

Z

z- spring, 26

About This Book

SORT Programme
A Structured Orthodontic Residents' Training Programme

A structured training programme is presented here, which is intended for any four-year postgraduate degree/ diploma in Orthodontics. A total of VIII modules have been developed, each of six months duration and the whole course is divided in these VIII modules. Its first four modules are structured in a way that they can be used for any two-years training programme.

The programme has been devised in a structured format, whereby, the whole training is patient-centered and follows the actual treatment sequence. Module-I is about activation of prior knowledge of basic medical and dental sciences and attainment of basic clinical knowledge and skills to prepare the residents for an empathetic patient care. Real patient encounter starts in Module-II and from here onwards, all areas of respective modules are according to treatment requirements at different stages. Each module has six distinct areas, i.e., Learning Objectives, Topics to be Covered, Reading List, Table of Specifications, Assessment Methods and Check List.

After successful adoption of this modular form of teaching, residents should attain the appropriate knowledge, proper attitudes and basic skills of orthodontics. This programme also enables the resident to develop a sense of professionalism, knowledge about medical ethics, scientific attitude, an inquisitive mind and a quest for research and Continuing Professional Development. A modular form of postgraduate training in orthodontics is suggested with an intention to standardize Orthodontic training across the country.